# Cross-Sectional Anatomy to Color and Study

Ray Poritsky, Ph.D.
Department of Anatomy
Case Western Reserve University
Cleveland, Ohio

**HANLEY & BELFUS, INC.,** Medical Publishers / Philadelphia
**MOSBY** / St. Louis • Baltimore • Boston • Carlsbad • Chicago • London • Madrid
• Naples • New York • Philadelphia • Sydney • Tokyo • Toronto

Publisher:      **HANLEY & BELFUS, INC.**
                Medical Publishers
                210 South 13th Street
                Philadelphia, PA 19107
                215/546-7293, 800/962-1892
                FAX 215/790-9330

North American and worldwide sales and distribution:

                **MOSBY**
                11830 Westline Industrial Drive
                St. Louis, MO 63146

In Canada:      Times Mirror Professional Publishing, Ltd.
                130 Flaska Drive
                Markham, Ontario L6G 1B8
                Canada

**Library of Congress Cataloging-in-Publication Data**

Poritsky, Raphael.
   Cross-sectional anatomy to color and study / Ray Poritsky.
      p.      cm.
   ISBN 1-56053-169-X (softcover : alk. paper)
   1. Anatomy, Surgical and topographical—Atlases.  2. Tomography—Atlases.
      3. Coloring books.  I. Title.
   [DNLM:  1. Anatomy, Regional—atlases.  2. Teaching Materials—atlases.
      3. Tomography—atlases.  QS 17 P836c 1996]
   QM531.P67  1996
   611' .0022'2 —dc20
   DNLM/DLC
   for Library of Congress                                        96-2015
                                                                      CIP

**CROSS-SECTIONAL ANATOMY TO COLOR AND STUDY**      ISBN 1-56053-169-X

Last digit is the print number:  9 8 7 6 5 4 3 2 1

# Introduction

The body sections in this book are presented in horizontal planes. The head is shown in both horizontal and coronal (frontal) planes. These planes are commonly used today by radiologists.

Due to the large number of anatomical structures in each section, paired structures (such as the kidney) are labeled on one side only. As the human body is bilaterally symmetrical (that is, one side is the mirror of the other), you will find the corresponding paired structure on the other side of the drawing in roughly the same position.

Keep in mind that all of the horizontal sections are drawn as if you are looking up from below. This is now the way MRIs and CT scans portray the body in cross section.

I have included some midsagittal (median) and three-dimensional drawings for orientation and to reinforce the reader's knowledge of anatomy. You may enjoy a few light moments over my cartoons, some etymological and some nonsensical, which I've included throughout this rather heavy subject matter.

The usual colors in anatomical illustrations are red for arteries, blue for veins, yellow for nerves, pink for muscles, and white or tan for bone. I hope that by coloring and labeling the drawings, the reader's knowledge of cross-sectional anatomy will be augmented and more easily remembered.

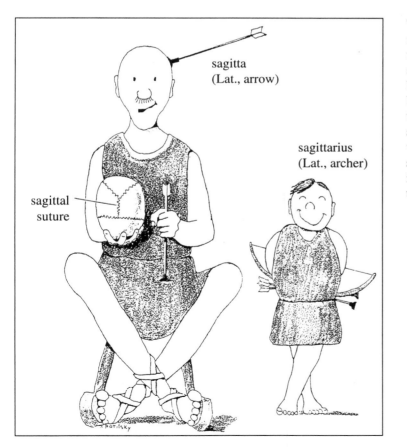

sagitta
(Lat., arrow)

sagittarius
(Lat., archer)

sagittal
suture

**The sagittal plane in anatomy** takes its name from the sagittal suture on the top of the skull. This suture is an interlocking seam that runs between the two parietal bones in a front-to-back direction. At the back of the skull, the sagittal suture meets the inverted V-shape of the lambdoid suture. With a bit of imagining, one can visualize the sagittal suture forming the shaft of an arrow and the adjacent diverging portions of the lamboid suture forming the feathers.

## Acknowledgments

I thank my colleague Dr. Barbara Freeman for her invaluable comments, suggestions, and criticism.

The following texts were used as references and source material: Dudley Morton, *Manual of Cross Section Anatomy*, The Williams & Wilkins Company, Baltimore, 1944; A. C. Eycleshymer and Tom Jones, *Hand-Atlas of Clinical Anatomy*, Lea & Febiger, Philadelphia, 1925; Spalteholz and Spanner, *Atlas of Systematic Human Anatomy*, 16th ed., F.A. Davis, Philadelphia, 1961; Harold Ellis, Bari Logan, and Adrian Dixon, *Human Cross-Sectional Anatomy*, Butterworth and Heinemann, Oxford, 1991; Walter Bo, Isadore Meschan, and Wayne Krueger, *Basic Atlas of Cross-Sectional Anatomy*, W.B. Saunders Company, Philadelphia, 1980; Frank Netter, *The Ciba Collection of Medical Illustrations*, Ciba Pharmaceutical Company, Summit, NJ, 1962; Carmine Clemente, *Anatomy: A Regional Atlas of the Human Body*, Urban & Schwarzenberg, Baltimore, 1987; G. Wolf-Heidegger, *Atlas of Systemic Human Anatomy*, Hafner Publishing Company, New York, 1962.

I did the drawings of the horizontal and coronal sections. The coronal head, neck, thorax, abdomen, and pelvis sections are preserved in plastic by the Sarcosote Company of Louisville, Kentucky and are used in teaching cross-sectional anatomy at the Case Western Reserve Medical School. The horizontal head drawings are based on colored photographs purchased from the Nasco Biological Supply Company of Fort Atkinson, Wisconsin. Sources for the drawings of the arm and leg are cited in the text. None of the drawings are exact replicas of the originals; modifications were made for the sake of clarity. Many of the drawings and cartoons are from my 1989 book *Anatomy to Color and Study*.

## I dedicate this book to my wife, Connie.

# Cross-Sectional Anatomy To Color and Study

## Table of Contents
*Structures listed represent approximate levels.*

# Cross-Sectional Anatomy To Color and Study

## Table of Contents (continued)
*Structures listed represent approximate levels.*

* In anatomy, the arm (Lat., brachium) extends from the shoulder to the elbow. The forearm (Lat., antebrachium) extends from the elbow to the wrist (Lat., carpus).

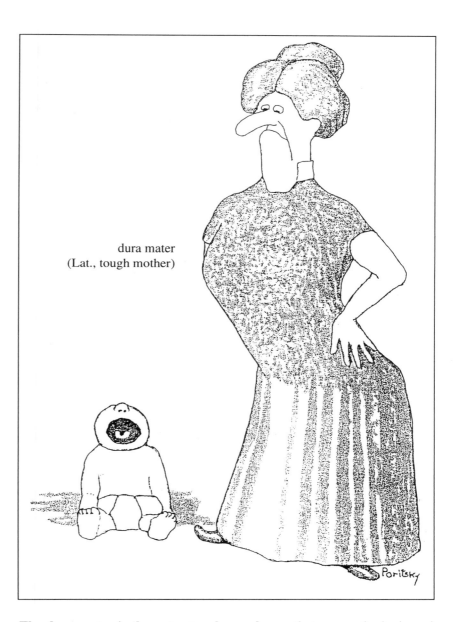

dura mater
(Lat., tough mother)

**The dura mater is the outer tough membrane** that covers the brain and spinal cord. This may seem an odd use of the phrase "tough mother," until one realizes that *dura mater* is a literal translation of the Arabic term into medieval Latin. The Arabs were fond of describing things in terms of family members. Here "mother" is used in the sense of "tough protector."

*Color and label:*

1. Scalp
2. Calvaria of skull
3. Diploë (spongy marrow of cranial bones)
4. Superior sagittal sinus (cut to show opening of superior cerebral vein)
5. Falx cerebri
6. Inferior sagittal sinus
7. Crista galli
8. Straight sinus
9. Great cerebral vein
10. Confluence of sinuses
11. Aperture of right transverse sinus
12. Occipital sinus
13. Falx cerebelli
14. Frontal sinus
15. Corpus callosum
16. Anterior cerebral artery
17. Septum pellucidum
18. Fornix
19. Thalamus and interthalamic adhesion
20. Optic chiasm
21. Pituitary gland (hypophysis)
22. Sphenoidal sinus
23. Mamillary body
24. Midbrain (mesencephalon)
25. Mesencephalic tectum
26. Pineal gland
27. Cerebral aqueduct
28. Cerebellum
29. Fourth ventricle
30. Cisterna magna (cerebellomedullary cistern)
31. Basilar artery
32. Left vertebral artery
33. Pons
34. Medulla oblongata
35. Spinal cord
36. Anterior arch of atlas
37. Body and dens of atlas
38. Pharyngeal tonsil
39. Ostium (opening) of auditory (eustachian) tube
40. Nasal pharynx
41. Middle nasal concha
42. Inferior nasal concha
43. Hard palate
44. Soft palate and uvula
45. Mandible
46. Hyoid bone
47. Genioglossus muscle
48. Geniohyoid muscle
49. Mylohyoid muscle
50. Epiglottis
51. Thyroid cartilage
52. Cricoid cartilage (arch and lamina)
53. Trachea
54. Oral pharynx
55. Laryngeal pharynx
56. Esophagus

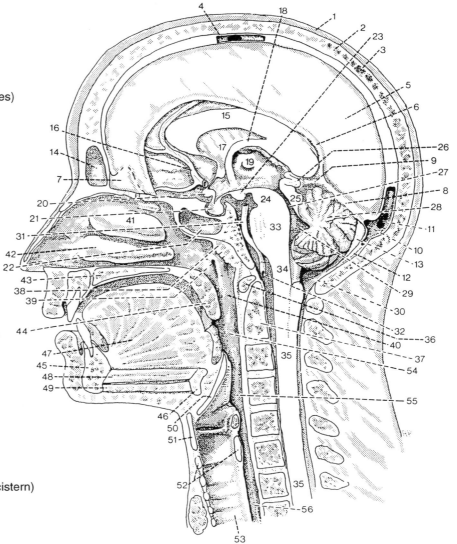

## Head and Neck, Midsagittal Aspect

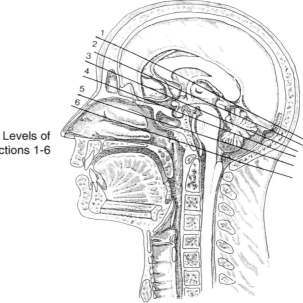

Levels of
Sections 1-6

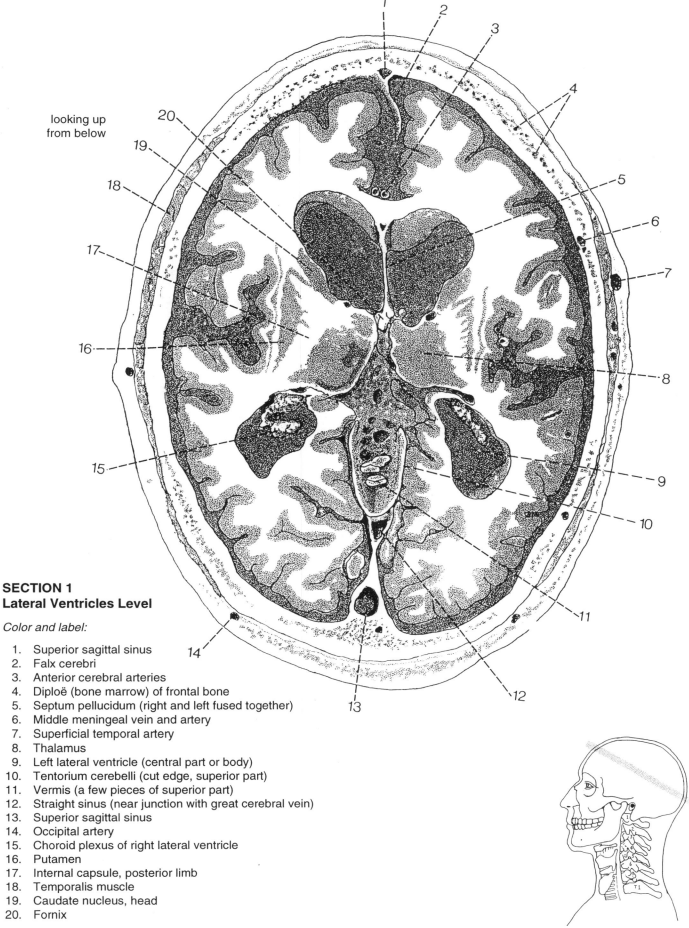

looking up
from below

**SECTION 1**
**Lateral Ventricles Level**

*Color and label:*

1.   Superior sagittal sinus
2.   Falx cerebri
3.   Anterior cerebral arteries
4.   Diploë (bone marrow) of frontal bone
5.   Septum pellucidum (right and left fused together)
6.   Middle meningeal vein and artery
7.   Superficial temporal artery
8.   Thalamus
9.   Left lateral ventricle (central part or body)
10.  Tentorium cerebelli (cut edge, superior part)
11.  Vermis (a few pieces of superior part)
12.  Straight sinus (near junction with great cerebral vein)
13.  Superior sagittal sinus
14.  Occipital artery
15.  Choroid plexus of right lateral ventricle
16.  Putamen
17.  Internal capsule, posterior limb
18.  Temporalis muscle
19.  Caudate nucleus, head
20.  Fornix

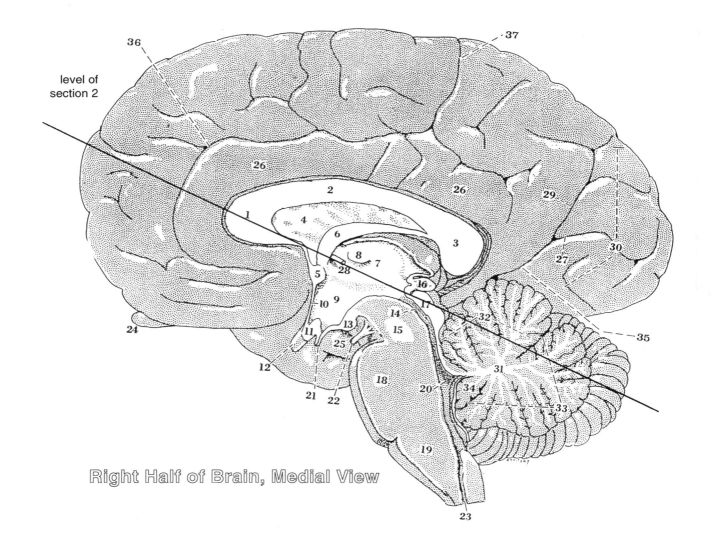

level of
section 2

Right Half of Brain, Medial View

*Color and label:*

1.  Genu of corpus callosum
2.  Body of corpus callosum
3.  Splenium of corpus callosum
4.  Septum pellucidum
5.  Anterior commissure
6.  Fornix
7.  Thalamus
8.  Interthalamic adhesion
9.  Hypothalamus
10. Lamina terminalis
11. Optic chiasm
12. Optic nerve
13. Mamillary body
14. Cerebral aqueduct
15. Decussation of the brachium conjunctivum
16. Pineal body
17. Mesencephalic tectum, formerly lamina quadrigemina
18. Pons
19. Medulla

20. Fourth ventricle
21. Infundibulum
22. Oculomotor nerve
23. Central canal of spinal cord
24. Olfactory bulb
25. Uncus on temporal lobe
26. Cingulate gyrus
27. Calcarine sulcus
28. Probe in interventricular foramen
29. Parieto-occipital sulcus
30. Occipital lobe
31. White matter of vermis
32. Anterior lobe of cerebellum
33. Posterior lobe of cerebellum
34. Nodulus of cerebellum
35. Common stem of parieto-occipital sulcus
    and calcarine sulcus
36. Cingulate sulcus
37. Marginal part of cingulate sulcus

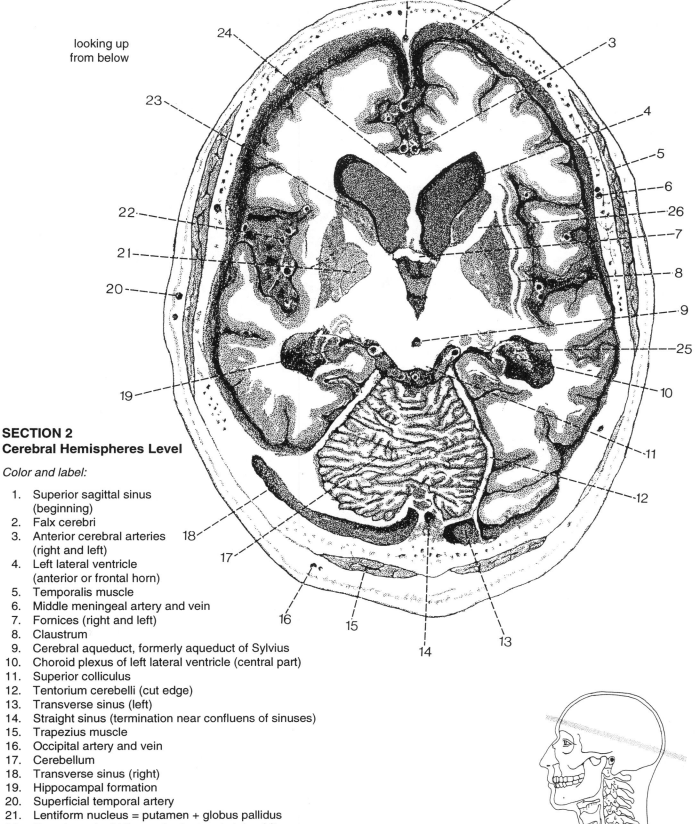

looking up
from below

## SECTION 2
## Cerebral Hemispheres Level

*Color and label:*

1. Superior sagittal sinus (beginning)
2. Falx cerebri
3. Anterior cerebral arteries (right and left)
4. Left lateral ventricle (anterior or frontal horn)
5. Temporalis muscle
6. Middle meningeal artery and vein
7. Fornices (right and left)
8. Claustrum
9. Cerebral aqueduct, formerly aqueduct of Sylvius
10. Choroid plexus of left lateral ventricle (central part)
11. Superior colliculus
12. Tentorium cerebelli (cut edge)
13. Transverse sinus (left)
14. Straight sinus (termination near confluens of sinuses)
15. Trapezius muscle
16. Occipital artery and vein
17. Cerebellum
18. Transverse sinus (right)
19. Hippocampal formation
20. Superficial temporal artery
21. Lentiform nucleus = putamen + globus pallidus
22. Branches of middle cerebral artery in lateral fissure
23. Caudate nucleus (head, uniting with putamen)
24. Genu of corpus callosum
25. Fimbria of hippocampus (beginning of fornix)
26. Anterior limb of internal capsule

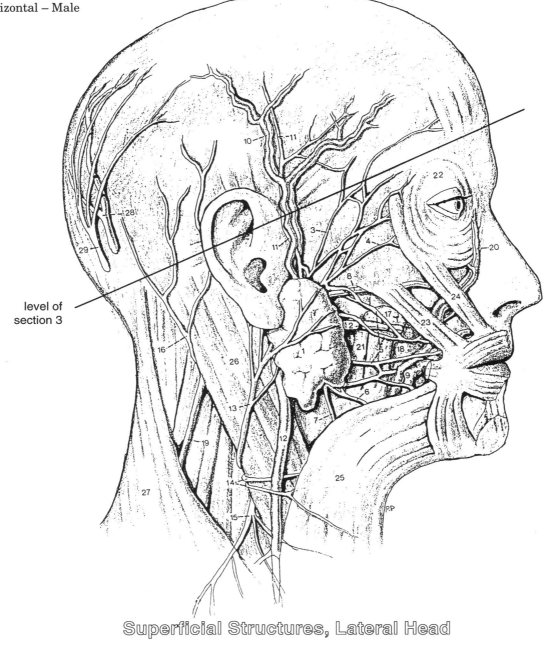

level of
section 3

Superficial Structures, Lateral Head

*Color and label:*

1. Parotid gland
2. Parotid duct
3. Temporal branches of facial nerve (VII)
4. Zygomatic branches of facial nerve (VII)
5. Buccal branches of facial nerve (VII)
6. Marginal mandibular branch of facial nerve (VII)
7. Cervical branch of facial nerve (VII)
8. Transverse facial artery
9. Facial artery and vein
10. Superficial temporal artery and vein
11. Auriculotemporal nerve
    (branch of mandibular nerve V3)
12. External jugular vein
13. Great auricular nerve
14. Transverse cervical nerve(s)

15. Supraclavicular nerves
16. Lesser occipital nerve
17. Accessory parotid gland
18. Buccal fat pad
19. Accessory nerve (XI)
20. Angular artery and vein
21. Masseter muscle
22. Orbicularis oculi
23. Zygomaticus major muscle
24. Zygomaticus minor muscle
25. Platysma muscle
26. Sternocleidomastoid muscle
27. Trapezius muscle
28. Occipital artery
29. Greater occipital nerve

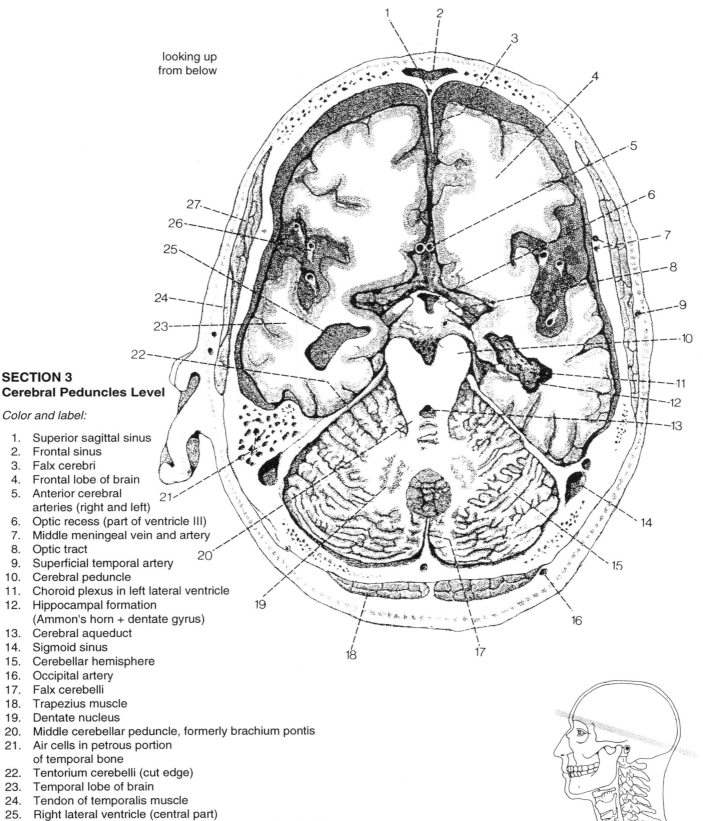

looking up
from below

**SECTION 3
Cerebral Peduncles Level**

*Color and label:*

1. Superior sagittal sinus
2. Frontal sinus
3. Falx cerebri
4. Frontal lobe of brain
5. Anterior cerebral
   arteries (right and left)
6. Optic recess (part of ventricle III)
7. Middle meningeal vein and artery
8. Optic tract
9. Superficial temporal artery
10. Cerebral peduncle
11. Choroid plexus in left lateral ventricle
12. Hippocampal formation
    (Ammon's horn + dentate gyrus)
13. Cerebral aqueduct
14. Sigmoid sinus
15. Cerebellar hemisphere
16. Occipital artery
17. Falx cerebelli
18. Trapezius muscle
19. Dentate nucleus
20. Middle cerebellar peduncle, formerly brachium pontis
21. Air cells in petrous portion
    of temporal bone
22. Tentorium cerebelli (cut edge)
23. Temporal lobe of brain
24. Tendon of temporalis muscle
25. Right lateral ventricle (central part)
26. Branches of middle cerebral artery in lateral (Sylvian) fissure
27. Temporalis muscle

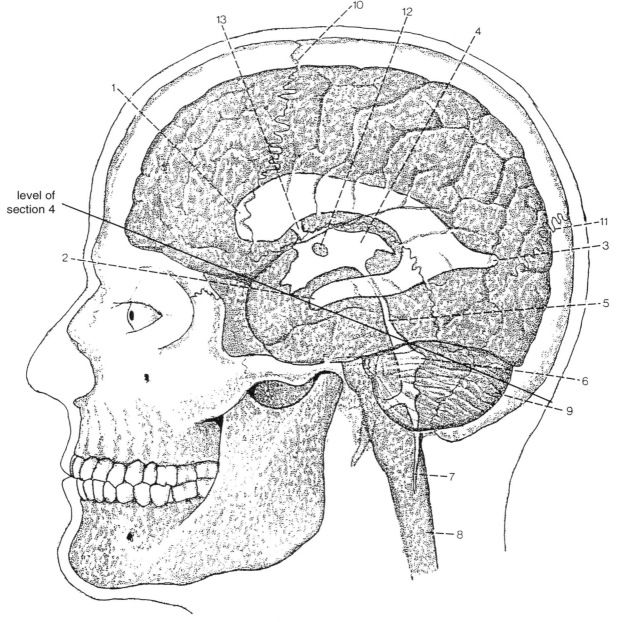

level of
section 4

Ventricles of the Brain in Relation to the Skull

*Color and label:*

1. Frontal (anterior) horn of lateral ventricle
2. Temporal (inferior) horn of lateral ventricle
3. Occipital (posterior) horn of lateral ventricle
4. Third ventricle
5. Cerebral aqueduct
6. Fourth ventricle
7. Central canal of spinal cord
8. Spinal cord
9. Cerebellum
10. Coronal suture
11. Lambdoid suture
12. Site of interthalamic adhesion
13. Interventricular foramen (of Monro)

looking up
from below

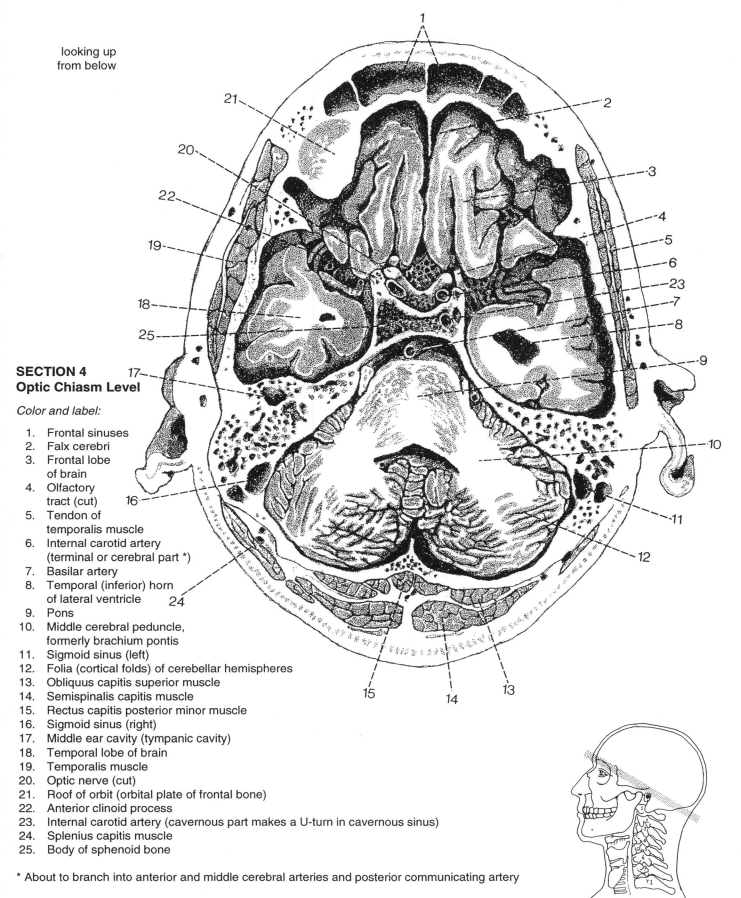

**SECTION 4**
**Optic Chiasm Level**

*Color and label:*

1. Frontal sinuses
2. Falx cerebri
3. Frontal lobe
   of brain
4. Olfactory
   tract (cut)
5. Tendon of
   temporalis muscle
6. Internal carotid artery
   (terminal or cerebral part *)
7. Basilar artery
8. Temporal (inferior) horn
   of lateral ventricle
9. Pons
10. Middle cerebral peduncle,
    formerly brachium pontis
11. Sigmoid sinus (left)
12. Folia (cortical folds) of cerebellar hemispheres
13. Obliquus capitis superior muscle
14. Semispinalis capitis muscle
15. Rectus capitis posterior minor muscle
16. Sigmoid sinus (right)
17. Middle ear cavity (tympanic cavity)
18. Temporal lobe of brain
19. Temporalis muscle
20. Optic nerve (cut)
21. Roof of orbit (orbital plate of frontal bone)
22. Anterior clinoid process
23. Internal carotid artery (cavernous part makes a U-turn in cavernous sinus)
24. Splenius capitis muscle
25. Body of sphenoid bone

\* About to branch into anterior and middle cerebral arteries and posterior communicating artery

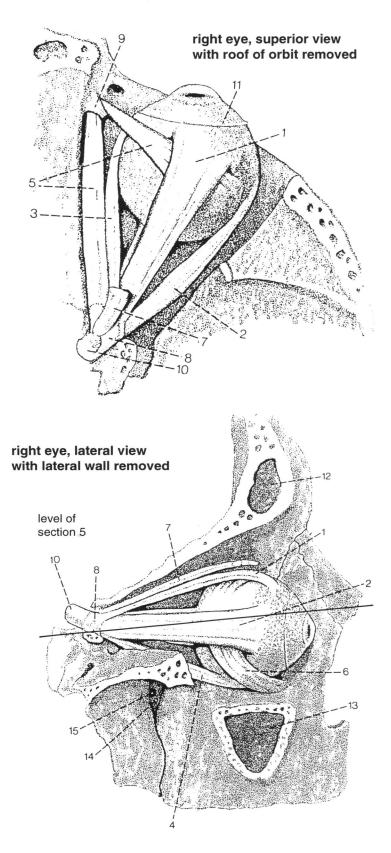

**right eye, superior view
with roof of orbit removed**

**right eye, lateral view
with lateral wall removed**

level of
section 5

Extraocular Muscles

*after Wolf-Heidegger*

*Color and label (at left):*

1. Superior rectus muscle
2. Lateral rectus muscle
3. Medial rectus muscle
4. Inferior rectus muscle
5. Superior oblique muscle
6. Inferior oblique muscle
7. Levator palpebrae muscle (cut)
8. Anulus tendineus communis
9. Trochlea
10. Optic nerve
11. Conjunctiva (tunica conjunctiva–cut edge)
12. Frontal sinus
13. Maxillary sinus
14. Pterygopalatine fossa
15. Sphenopalatine foramen

## SECTION 5
## Eye, Nasal Sinuses Level

*Color and label (at right):*

1. Frontal sinus
2. Frontalis belly of occipitofrontalis muscle
3. Superior portion of left eye
4. Lacrimal gland
5. Orbital fat
6. Ethmoid air cells
7. Optic nerve of left eye ensheathed by three meninges
8. Sphenoid sinus
9. Tendon of temporalis muscle
10. Internal carotid artery (cut posteriorly entering and anteriorly exiting cavernous sinus)
11. Superficial temporal artery and vein
12. Basilar artery
13. Cochlea
14. Pons (inferior aspect), abducent nerve (cranial nerve VI)
15. Air cells in petrous portion of temporal bone
16. Sigmoid sinus (left)
17. Cerebellar hemisphere
18. Splenius capitis muscle
19. Medulla oblongata, pyramids (ventrally)
20. Semispinalis capitis
21. Rectus capitis posterior minor muscle

*Continued...*

looking up
from below

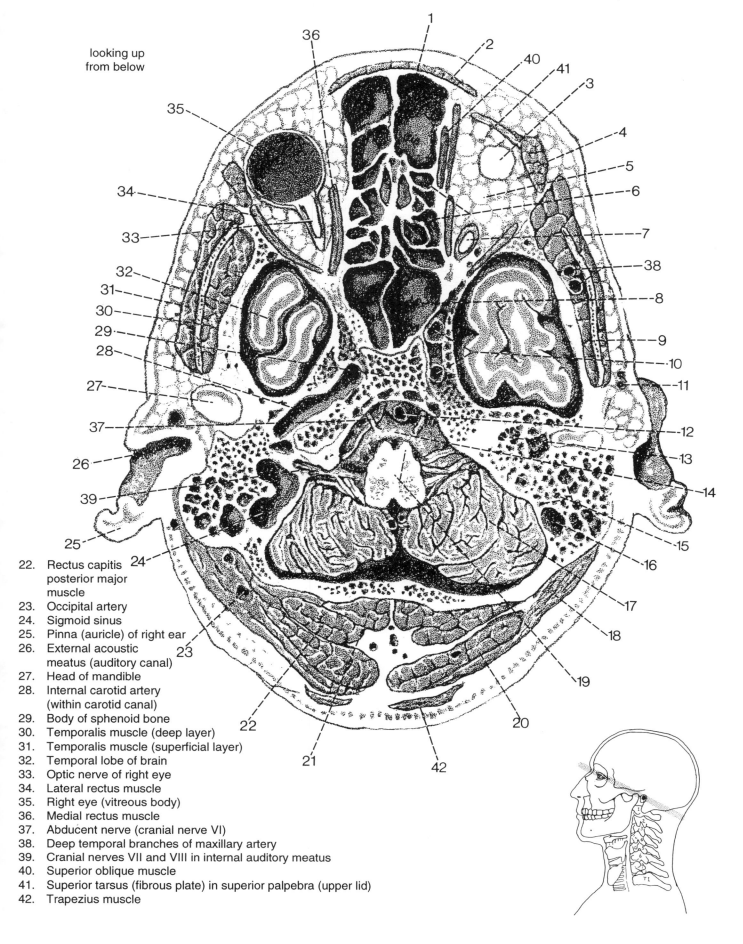

22. Rectus capitis
    posterior major
    muscle
23. Occipital artery
24. Sigmoid sinus
25. Pinna (auricle) of right ear
26. External acoustic
    meatus (auditory canal)
27. Head of mandible
28. Internal carotid artery
    (within carotid canal)
29. Body of sphenoid bone
30. Temporalis muscle (deep layer)
31. Temporalis muscle (superficial layer)
32. Temporal lobe of brain
33. Optic nerve of right eye
34. Lateral rectus muscle
35. Right eye (vitreous body)
36. Medial rectus muscle
37. Abducent nerve (cranial nerve VI)
38. Deep temporal branches of maxillary artery
39. Cranial nerves VII and VIII in internal auditory meatus
40. Superior oblique muscle
41. Superior tarsus (fibrous plate) in superior palpebra (upper lid)
42. Trapezius muscle

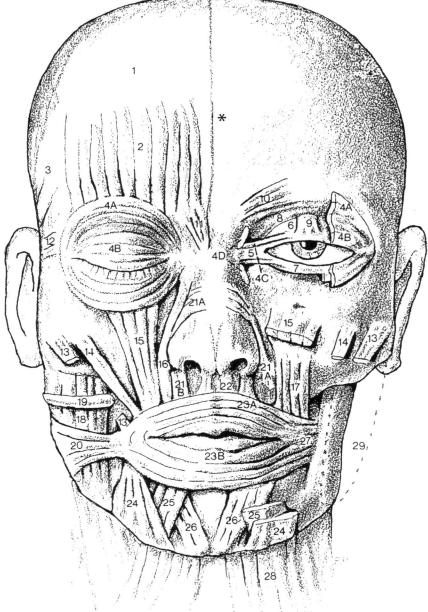

Muscles of Facial Expression

*Color and label\*:*

1. Galea aponeurotica, cut edge (epicranial aponeurosis)
2. Frontal belly of occipitofrontalis
3. Temporoparietalis
4. Orbicularis oculi
   *A*, orbital part    *B*, palpebral part
   *C*, lacrimal part   *D*, origin of orbital part
5. Medial palpebral ligament
6. Superior tarsus of eyelid
7. Inferior tarsus of eyelid
8. Orbital septum
9. Tendon of levator palpebrae
10. Corrugator supercilii
11. Procerus
12. Auricularis anterior
13. Zygomaticus major
14. Zygomaticus minor

15. Levator labii superioris (Lat., raiser of the superior lip)
16. Levator labii superioris alaeque nasi
17. Levator anguli oris
18. Masseter
19. Parotid duct
20. Risorius
21. Nasalis   *A*, transverse part *B*, alar part
22. Depressor septi
23. Orbicularis oris   *A*, marginal part *B*, labial part
24. Depressor anguli oris
    (Lat., depressor of the mouth angle)
25. Depressor labii inferioris
26. Mentalis
27. Buccinator (Lat., trumpeter)
28. Platysma
29. Outline of the masseter

\* All of these muscles, except the masseter, are innervated by the facial nerve.

looking up
from below

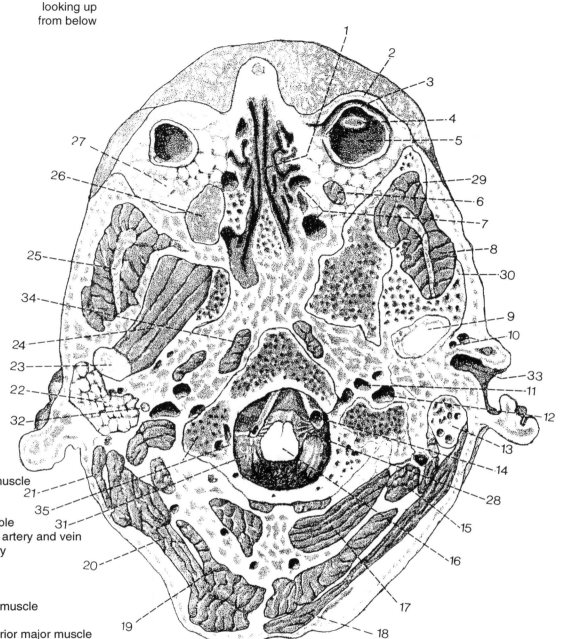

**SECTION 6**
**Nasal Cavity Level**

*Color and label:*

1. Nasal septum
   (perpindicular plate
   of ethmoid bone)
2. Palpebra superioris
   (upper lid)
3. Cornea
4. Lens of eye
5. Vitreous body
6. Inferior rectus eye muscle
7. Ethmoid air cells
8. Temporalis muscle
9. Head (left) of mandible
10. Superficial temporal artery and vein
11. Internal carotid artery
12. Internal jugular vein
13. Mastoid process
14. Vertebral artery
15. Longissimus capitis muscle
16. Medulla oblongata
17. Rectus capitis posterior major muscle
18. Trapezius muscle
19. Semispinalis capitis
20. Sternocleidomastoid muscle
21. Splenius capitis muscle
22. Parotid gland
23. Head (right) of mandible
24. Lateral pterygoid muscle
25. Tendon of temporalis muscle
26. Roof (apex) of maxillary sinus
27. Fat of right orbit
28. Rootlets of nerve XII (hypoglossal)
29. Temporal process of zygomatic bone (anterior part of zygomatic arch)
30. Zygomatic process of temporal bone (posterior part of zygomatic arch)
31. Tonsil of cerebellum
32. Facial nerve (N VII) in facial canal
33. External acoustic meatus (ear canal)
34. Rectus capitis anterior muscle
35. Basilar part of occipital bone and margin of foramen magnum

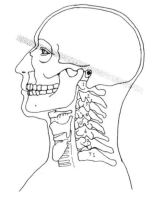

## SECTION 7
## Mastoid Air Cells Level

*Color and label:*

1. Naris (Lat., nostril; pl. nares)
2. Maxillary sinus
3. Inferior nasal concha
4. Nasal cavity
5. Coronoid process of mandible
6. Vomer bone (part of nasal septum)
7. Lingual nerve (branch of mandibular nerve)
8. Inferior alveolar nerve (branch of mandibular nerve)
9. Neck of mandible
10. External carotid artery
11. External auditory meatus
12. Cartilage in pinna of ear
13. Styloid process
14. Jugular foramen (beginning of internal jugular vein)
15. Splenius capitis muscle
16. Vertebral artery
17. Pyramids of medulla oblongata
18. Semispinalis capitis muscle
19. Cerebellum

20. Sigmoid sinus
21. Mastoid air cells
22. Facial nerve
23. Internal carotid artery
24. Parotid gland
25. Lateral pterygoid muscle
26. Auditory (eustachian) tube
27. Temporalis muscle and tendon
28. Maxilla (zygomatic process)
29. Glossopharyngeal nerve (IX), vagus nerve (X), accessory nerve (XI) just medial to jugular foramen
30. Neck of mandible
31. Hypoglossal nerve (cranial nerve XII)
32. Masseter muscle
33. Maxillary artery
34. Longus capitis muscle
35. Pharyngeal tubercle of occipital bone
36. External carotid artery and retromandibular vein
37. Medial pterygoid muscle

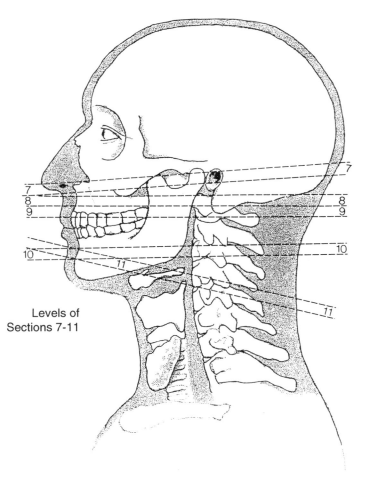

Levels of
Sections 7-11

looking up
from below

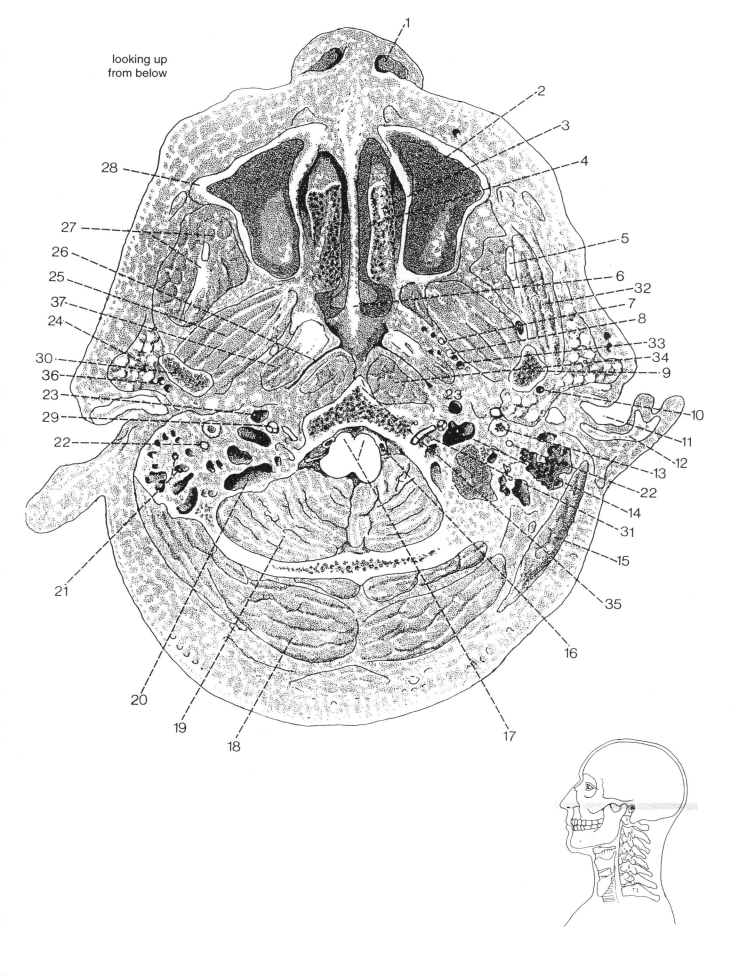

Brain, Inferior View

Color and label (above):

1. Olfactory bulb
2. Olfactory tract
3. Olfactory trigone
4. Medial olfactory stria
5. Lateral olfactory stria
6. Anterior perforated substance
7. Optic nerve (II)
8. Optic chiasma
9. Optic tract
10. Infundibulum
11. Tuber cinereum
12. Mamillary body
13. Cerebral peduncle
14. Uncus
15. Oculomotor nerve (III)
16. Pons
17. Trigeminal nerve (V)
18. Abducent nerve (VI)
19. Facial nerve (VII), motor
20. Nervus intermedius (part of facial nerve, VII)
21. Vestibulocochlear nerve (VIII)
22. Glossopharyngeal nerve (IX)
23. Vagus nerve (X)
24. Accessory nerve (XI)
25. Pyramids
26. Hypoglossal nerve (XII)
27. Cerebellum (hemisphere)
28. Trochlear nerve (IV)

## SECTION 8
## Maxillary Sinus Level

Color and label (at right):

1. Mucosa of hard palate
2. Orbicularis oris muscle
3. Vestibule of mouth (space between cheek and teeth/gums)
4. Maxilla
5. Buccinator muscle
6. Palatine glands
7. Temporalis muscle
8. Medial pterygoid muscle
9. Ramus of mandible
10. Nasopharynx (narrow space) lined with surrounding mucosa and wall formed by superior pharyngeal constrictor muscle (posteriorly and laterally)
11. Parotid gland
12. Retromandibular vein (lateral) and external carotid artery (medial)

Continued...

looking up
from below

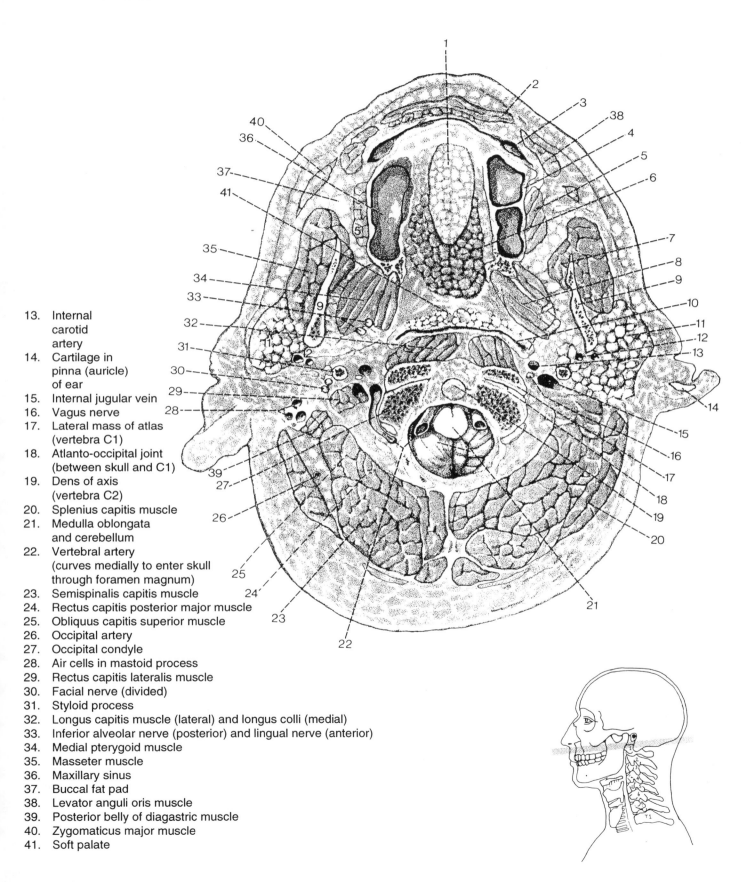

13. Internal
    carotid
    artery
14. Cartilage in
    pinna (auricle)
    of ear
15. Internal jugular vein
16. Vagus nerve
17. Lateral mass of atlas
    (vertebra C1)
18. Atlanto-occipital joint
    (between skull and C1)
19. Dens of axis
    (vertebra C2)
20. Splenius capitis muscle
21. Medulla oblongata
    and cerebellum
22. Vertebral artery
    (curves medially to enter skull
    through foramen magnum)
23. Semispinalis capitis muscle
24. Rectus capitis posterior major muscle
25. Obliquus capitis superior muscle
26. Occipital artery
27. Occipital condyle
28. Air cells in mastoid process
29. Rectus capitis lateralis muscle
30. Facial nerve (divided)
31. Styloid process
32. Longus capitis muscle (lateral) and longus colli (medial)
33. Inferior alveolar nerve (posterior) and lingual nerve (anterior)
34. Medial pterygoid muscle
35. Masseter muscle
36. Maxillary sinus
37. Buccal fat pad
38. Levator anguli oris muscle
39. Posterior belly of diagastric muscle
40. Zygomaticus major muscle
41. Soft palate

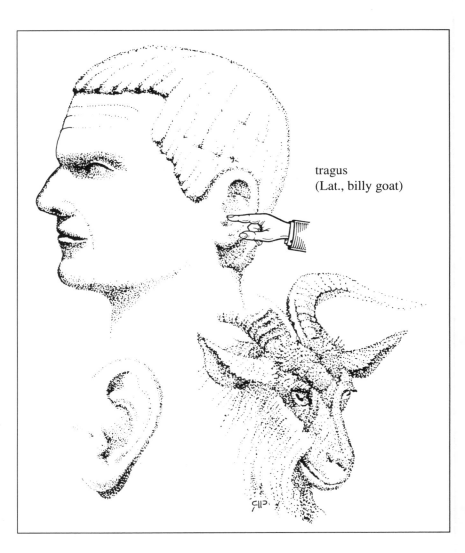

tragus
(Lat., billy goat)

**The tragus of the ear** was so named because in some old men it grows a little tuft of hair that reminded the ancient anatomists of a billy goat's beard. *Tragedy* originally meant "goat's song."

## SECTION 9
## Tongue, Teeth of Upper Jaw Level

*Color and label:*

1. Intrinsic tongue muscles
2. Orbicularis oris muscle
3. Teeth of upper jaw (roots in maxilla)
4. Buccinator muscle
5. Oral cavity
6. Masseter muscle
7. Ramus of mandible
8. Inferior alveolar nerve and artery
9. Styloid process
10. Internal carotid artery
11. Internal jugular vein
12. Vertebral artery
13. Lateral mass of atlas (vertebra C1)
14. Splenius capitis muscle
15. Occipital bone forming posterior rim of foramen magnum
16. Rectus capitis posterior major muscle
17. Semispinalis capitis muscle
18. Spinal cord
19. Obliquus capitis inferior muscle
20. Longissimus capitis muscle
21. Dens of axis
22. Rectus capitis lateralis muscle
23. Parotid gland

*Continued...*

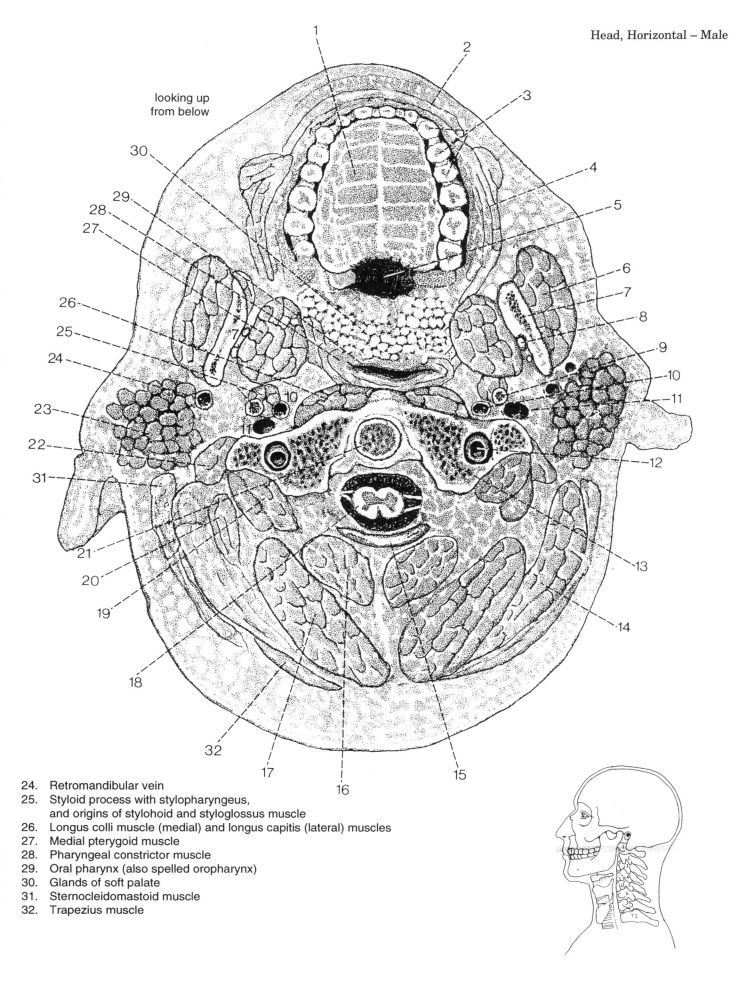

looking up
from below

24. Retromandibular vein
25. Styloid process with stylopharyngeus,
    and origins of stylohoid and styloglossus muscle
26. Longus colli muscle (medial) and longus capitis (lateral) muscles
27. Medial pterygoid muscle
28. Pharyngeal constrictor muscle
29. Oral pharynx (also spelled oropharynx)
30. Glands of soft palate
31. Sternocleidomastoid muscle
32. Trapezius muscle

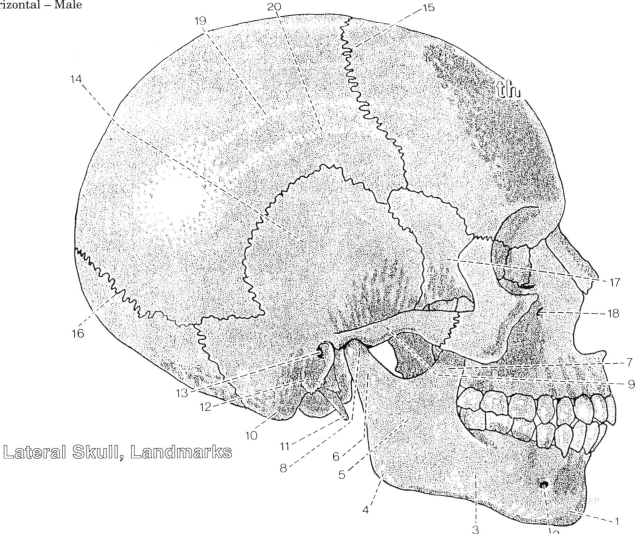

Lateral Skull, Landmarks

**SECTION 10**
**Mandible, Roots of Teeth Level**

*Color and label (at right):*

1. Roots of teeth in mandible (lower jaw)
2. Oribicularis oris muscle
3. Transverse intrinsic tongue muscles
4. Lingual nerve (branch of mandibular nerve)
5. Inferior alveolar nerve (branch of mandibular nerve) within mandibular canal
6. Ramus of mandible
7. Oral pharynx
8. Retromandibular vein
9. Parotid gland
10. Internal carotid artery
11. Internal jugular vein
12. Roots of cervical nerve C3 (ventral root above, posterior root below)
13. Semispinalis cervicis muscle
14. Trapezius muscle
15. Semispinalis capitis muscle
16. Splenius capitis muscle
17. Spinal cord
18. Vertebral artery
19. Sternocleidomastoid muscle
20. Body and transverse process of vertebra C3

*Continued...*

*Color and label (above):*

1. Mental protuberance
2. Mental foramen
3. Body of mandible
4. Angle of mandible
5. Ramus of mandible
6. Condyloid process
7. Coronoid process
8. Head of mandible
9. Zygomatic arch
10. Mastoid process
11. Styloid process
12. Tympanic part of temporal bone
13. External auditory meatus
14. Squamous part of temporal bone
15. Coronal suture
16. Lambdoid suture
17. Greater wing of sphenoid bone
18. Infraorbital foramen
19. Superior temporal line
20. Inferior temporal line

looking up
from below

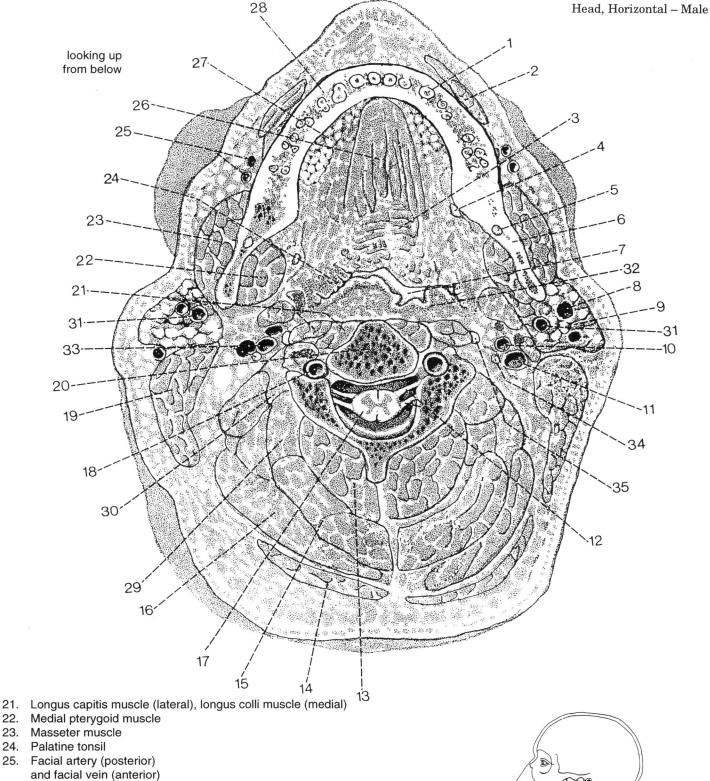

21. Longus capitis muscle (lateral), longus colli muscle (medial)
22. Medial pterygoid muscle
23. Masseter muscle
24. Palatine tonsil
25. Facial artery (posterior)
    and facial vein (anterior)
26. Genioglossus muscle
27. Sublingual gland
28. Mandible (body)
29. Levator scapulae muscle
30. Scalene muscles
31. External carotid artery
32. Pharyngeal constrictor muscle
33. Internal carotid artery (medial), internal jugular vein (lateral),
    and vagus nerve
34. Left vagus nerve
35. Sympathetic trunk

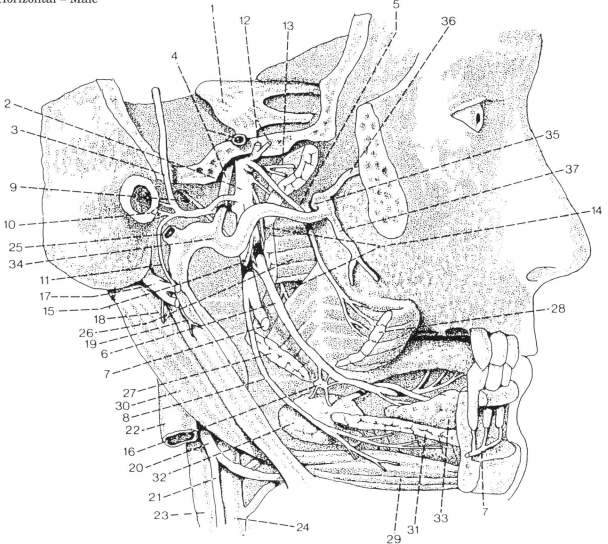

Mandibular Nerve, Maxillary Artery

*Color and label:*

1. Trigeminal ganglion
2. Mandibular nerve
3. Auriculotemporal nerve (note its two roots surrounding the middle meningeal artery)
4. Middle meningeal artery
5. Buccal nerve (sensory to mucous membrane and skin of cheek)
6. Lingual nerve (supplies general sensation to anterior two-thirds of tongue)
7. Inferior alveolar nerve (cut)
8. Mylohyoid nerve (motor to mylohyoid muscle and anterior belly of digastric muscle)
9. Chorda tympani (branch of facial nerve carrying taste fibers and parasympathetic fibers to lingual nerve; exits skull through petrotympanic fissure)
10. External acoustic meatus nerves
11. Communicating branch with facial nerve
12. Deep temporal nerves (motor to temporalis muscle)
13. Lateral pterygoid nerve
14. Medial pterygoid nerve
15. Masseteric nerve
16. Submandibular ganglion
17. Facial nerve

18. Digastric branch of facial nerve (motor to posterior belly of digastric muscle)
19. Stylohyoid branch of facial nerve
20. Hypoglossal nerve
21. Superior root of ansa cervicalis
22. Internal jugular vein
23. Internal carotid artery
24. External carotid artery
25. Superficial temporal artery (cut)
26. Lateral pterygoid muscle (cut)
27. Medial pterygoid muscle (cut)
28. Buccinator muscle (cut and reflected)
29. Anterior belly of digastric muscle
30. Posterior belly of digastric muscle
31. Mylohyoid muscle
32. Submandibular gland (note its duct crossing the lingual nerve)
33. Sublingual gland
34. Maxillary artery (most of its branches are not shown)
35. Sphenopalatine artery entering nasal cavity through sphenopalatine foramen
36. Infraorbital artery
37. Posterior superior alveolar artery

looking up
from below

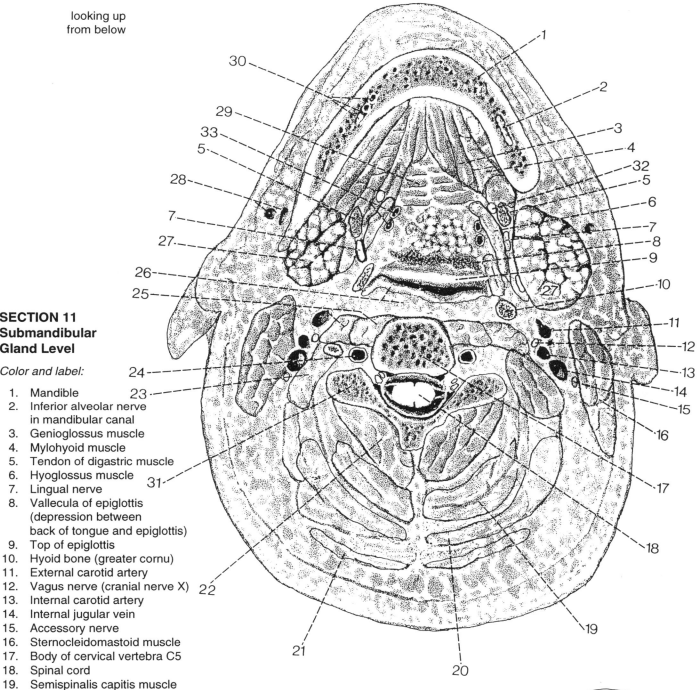

**SECTION 11
Submandibular
Gland Level**

*Color and label:*

1. Mandible
2. Inferior alveolar nerve
   in mandibular canal
3. Genioglossus muscle
4. Mylohyoid muscle
5. Tendon of digastric muscle
6. Hyoglossus muscle
7. Lingual nerve
8. Vallecula of epiglottis
   (depression between
   back of tongue and epiglottis)
9. Top of epiglottis
10. Hyoid bone (greater cornu)
11. External carotid artery
12. Vagus nerve (cranial nerve X)
13. Internal carotid artery
14. Internal jugular vein
15. Accessory nerve
16. Sternocleidomastoid muscle
17. Body of cervical vertebra C5
18. Spinal cord
19. Semispinalis capitis muscle
20. Splenius capitis muscle
21. Trapezius muscle
22. Multifidus muscle
23. Scalenus medius muscle
24. Vertebral artery
25. Longus capitis (lateral) and longus colli (medial) muscles
26. Pharyngeal constrictor muscle and oral pharynx (oropharynx)
27. Submandibular gland
28. Facial vein (superficial) and facial artery (deep)
29. Transverse intrinsic muscle of tongue
30. Inferior alveolar artery, vein, and nerve in mandibular canal
31. Transverse process of C5
32. Hypoglossal nerve (XII)
33. Lingual artery (anterior) and vein (posterior)

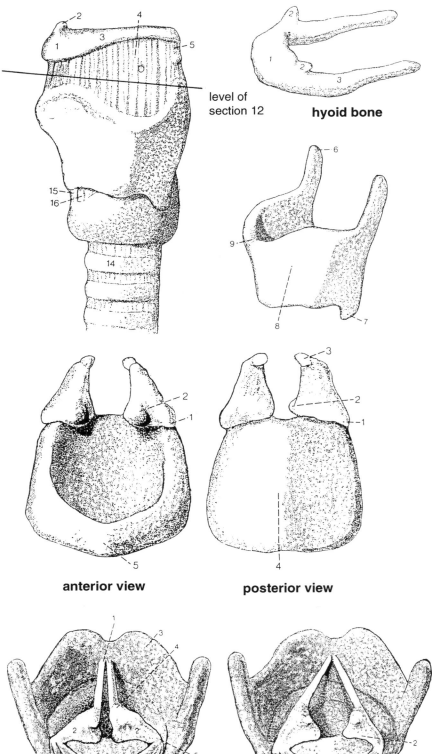

**hyoid bone**

**anterior view**

**posterior view**

**adduction**

**abduction**

**vocal ligaments**

## Larynx, Cartilages

*Color and label (at left):*

1. Body of hyoid bone
2. Lesser horn (cornu) of hyoid bone
3. Greater horn (cornu) of hyoid bone
4. Thyrohyoid membrane
5. Lateral thyrohyoid ligament
6. Superior horn of thyroid cartilage
7. Inferior horn of thyroid cartilage
8. Lamina of thyroid cartilage
9. Superior thyroid notch

(Numbers 10–14 are depicted at right)

10. Arytenoid cartilage
    (Gr., arytaina—pitcher, ladle)
11. Arch of cricoid cartilage
12. Lamina of cricoid cartilage
13. Facet for inferior horn of
    thyroid cartilage
14. Tracheal rings
15. Cricothyroid ligament
16. Conus elasticus

*Color and label (at left):*

1. Muscular process of arytenoid cartilage
2. Vocal process of arytenoid cartilage
3. Corniculate cartilage
4. Lamina of cricoid cartilage
5. Arch of cricoid cartilage

*Color and label (at left):*

1. Vocal ligaments
2. Arytenoid cartilage
3. Thyroid cartilage
4. Vocal process of arytenoid cartilage
5. Muscular process of arytenoid cartilage
6. Lamina of cricoid cartilage
7. Posterior cricoarytenoid muscle (by pulling
   the muscular processes of arytenoid
   cartilages posterior, the two vocal processes
   separate [abduct] and a diamond-shaped
   space [rima glottidis] opens between the two
   vocal ligaments)

level of
section 12

looking up
from below

**SECTION 12**
**Thyrohyoid**
**Membrane Level**

*Color and label:*

1. Thyrohyoid membrane
2. Sternohyoid muscle
3. Glosso-epiglottic fat pad
4. Omohyoid muscle
   (superior belly)
5. Aryepiglottic muscle in
   aryepiglottic fold
6. Laryngeal pharynx
   (laryngopharynx)
7. Inferior pharyngeal
   constrictor muscle
8. Common facial vein (joining
   internal jugular vein)
9. Common carotid artery
10. Sternocleidomastoid
    muscle
11. Internal jugular vein
12. Vagus nerve (X) (left)
13. Longus capitis muscle
14. Accessory nerve (XI)
15. Longus colli muscle
16. Scalenus medius muscle
17. Longissimus cervicis muscle
18. Levator scapulae muscle
19. Body of cervical vertebra C4
20. Deep cervical vein
21. Semispinalis capitis muscle
22. Splenius capitis (medial) and
    splenius cervicis (lateral) muscles
23. Trapezius muscle
24. Spinal cord and denticulate ligament
25. Ligamentum nuchae (nuchal ligament)
26. Bifid (doubled) spinous
    process of vertebra C4
27. Semispinalis cervicis muscle
28. Lamina and ligamentum
    flavum (yellow ligament)
29. Multifidus muscle
30. Dorsal root ganglion of
    fourth cervical nerve
31. Vertebral artery and vein
32. External jugular vein
33. Right internal jugular vein
34. Right vagus nerve
35. Right common carotid artery
36. Superior horn of thyroid cartilage
37. Right common facial vein
38. Piriform recess
39. Platysma muscle
40. Submandibular gland
41. Thyrohyoid muscle
42. Epiglottis - laryngeal surface (facing laryngeal inlet)
43. Epiglottic cartilage (cut)
44. Sympathetic trunk
45. Scalenus anterior muscle and phrenic nerve
46. Longissimus capitis muscle

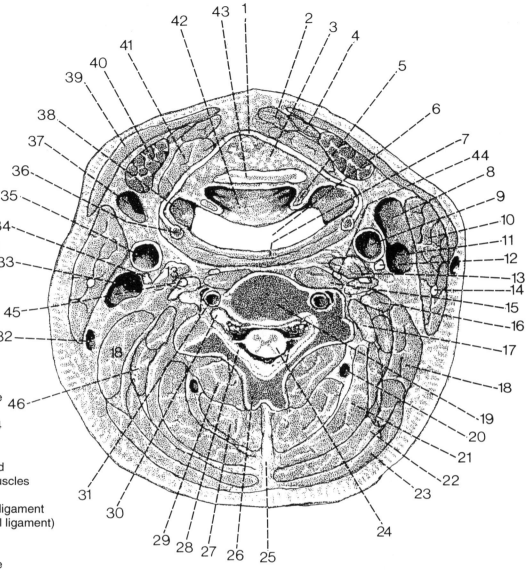

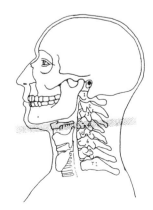

# Muscles of the Pharynx

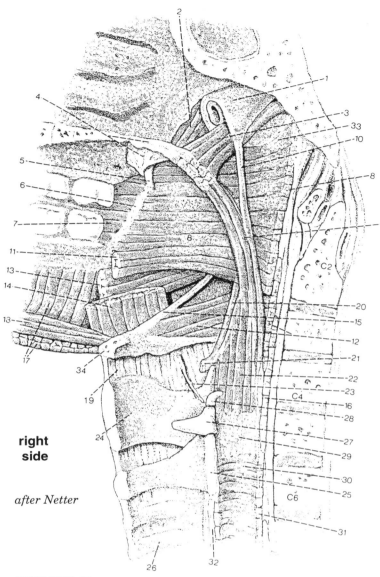

**right side**

*after Netter*

Color and label (at left):

1. Auditory tube (cartilaginous part)
2. Tensor veli palatini muscle
3. Levator veli palatini muscle
4. Tendon of tensor veli palatini and palatine aponeurosis
5. Hamulus of medial pterygoid plate
6. Pterygomandibular raphe
7. Buccinator muscle
8. Superior pharyngeal constrictor muscle
9. Palatopharyngeus muscle
10. Salpingopharyngeus muscle
11. Glossopharyngeus (of superior constrictor)
12. Middle pharyngeal constrictor muscle
13. Styloglossus muscle
14. Hyoglossus muscle
15. Stylohyoid ligament
16. Inferior constrictor
17. Mylohyoid muscle
18. Geniohyoid muscle
19. Thyrohyoid membrane
20. Stylopharyngeus muscle
21. Fibers to pharyngoepiglottic fold
22. Longitudinal muscle of pharynx
23. Internal branch of superior laryngeal nerve
24. Thyroid cartilage
25. Cricoid cartilage
26. Trachea
27. Arytenoid cartilage
28. Corniculate cartilage
29. Pharyngeal aponeurosis
30. Cricopharyngeus muscle (part of inferior constrictor)
31. Esophageal circular muscle
32. Esophageal longitudinal muscle
33. Pharyngobasilar fascia
34. Hyoid bone

## SECTION 13
## Vocal Cords, Rima Glottidis Level

Color and label (at right):

1. Vocalis muscle (lateral to vocal ligament)
2. Sternohyoid muscle
3. Thyroarytenoid muscle
4. Vocal ligament (formed by medial superior edge of conus elasticus; length of vocal cords or folds is rough ly 60% elastic ligament and 40% arytenoid cartilage)
5. Rima (Lat., slit) glottidis (space between vocal cords)
6. Omohyoid muscle (superior belly)
7. Lateral cricoarytenoid muscle
8. Arytenoid cartilage (muscular process)
9. Posterior cricoarytenoid muscle (this muscle is the only opener or abductor of the vocal cords)
10. Thyroid gland–left lobe, superior extension
11. Left common carotid artery
12. Sternocleidomastoid muscle
13. Internal jugular vein (left)
14. Vagus nerve (X)
15. Intervertebral disk between vertebra C4 and C5

16. Cervical nerves (anterior rami) forming brachial plexus
17. External jugular vein
18. Anterior and posterior tubercles of transverse process of vertebra C5
19. Dorsal root ganglion of 5th cervical nerve
20. Lateral mass of vertebra C6
21. Body of vertebra C5
22. Lamina of vertebra C6
23. Spinal cord
24. Interspinalis cervicis muscles (lateral) and interspinalis ligaments (medial)
25. Multifidus muscle
26. Vertebral artery and vein
27. Semispinalis cervicis muscle
28. Semispinalis capitis muscle
29. Splenius capitis muscle
30. Levator scapulae muscle

*Continued...*

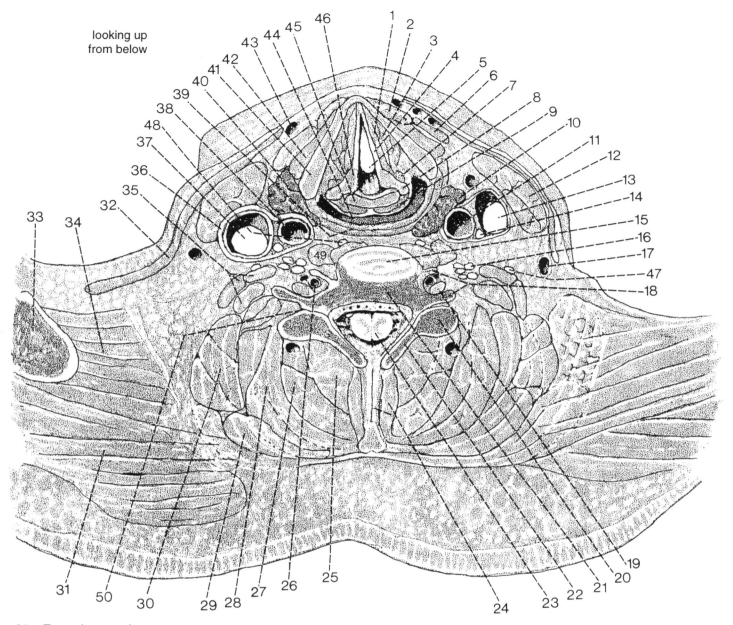

looking up
from below

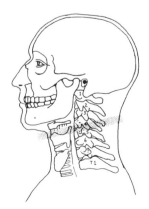

31. Trapezius muscle
32. Plastysma muscle
33. Clavicle
34. Trapezius muscle
35. Scalene muscles
36. Carotid sheath containing internal jugular vein,
    common carotid artery, and vagus nerve
37. Right internal jugular vein
38. Right common carotid artery
39. Inferior pharyngeal constrictor muscle
40. Thyroid gland (right lobe)
41. Thyroid cartilage (lamina)
42. Thyrohyoid muscle
43. Anterior jugular vein
44. Laryngeal pharynx (laryngopharynx)
45. Cricoid cartilage (lamina)
46. Arytenoid cartilage (vocal process)
47. Phrenic nerve, lying just in front of anterior scalene muscle
48. Sympathetic trunk, lying just anterior to longus colli muscle
49. Longus capitis muscle
50. Articulation (synovial joint) between inferior articular process of C5 and superior articular process of C6

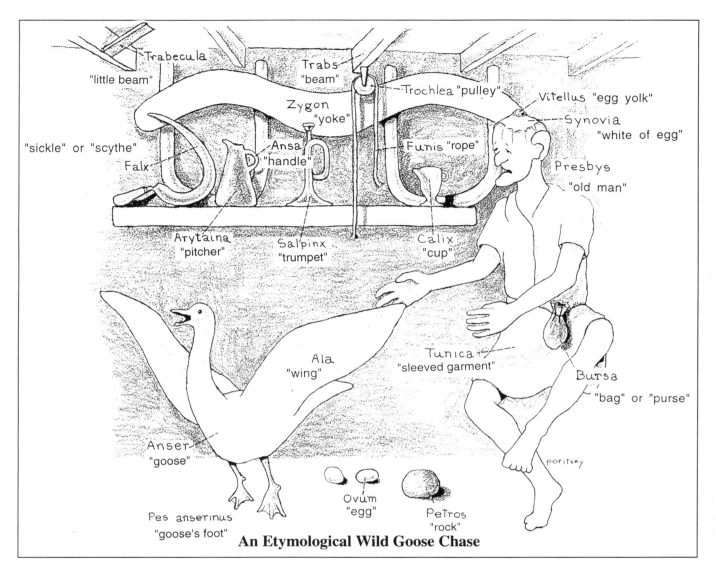

**An Etymological Wild Goose Chase**

Labels in figure: Trabecula "little beam"; Trabs "beam"; Trochlea "pulley"; Vitellus "egg yolk"; Zygon "yoke"; Synovia "white of egg"; "sickle" or "scythe"; Falx; Ansa "handle"; Funis "rope"; Presbys "old man"; Arytaina "pitcher"; Sal'pinx "trumpet"; Calix "cup"; Ala "wing"; Tunica "sleeved garment"; Bursa "bag" or "purse"; Anser "goose"; Pes anserinus "goose's foot"; Ovum "egg"; Petros "rock"; poritsky

**Anser** is "goose" in Latin and **pes anserinus** is "goose's foot."

**Presbys** is "old man" in Greek. Presbyterion is a council of elders. Presbyopia (literally "old eyes") is the loss of near vision that occurs with advancing age. Presbyacusis (literally "old hearing") is loss of hearing as part of the aging process.

**Ala** is "wing" in Latin. There's an ala in the nose, another in the ilium of the hip bone, and the sphenoid bone has two wings or alae–a greater wing and a lesser wing.

**Petros** is "rock" in Greek and is used for the hard "rocky" or petrous portion of the temporal bone. Peter means "rock."

**Tunica** in ancient Rome was an ordinary sleeved garment. In anatomy it is a name given to coats or coverings.

**Bursa** was a "bag" or "purse" in Latin and is derived from the Greek bursa–"a hide or wineskin." In medical parlance, a bursa is a flattened sac containing a slippery fluid that allows structures to slide smoothly past one another.

**Vitellus** meant "egg yolk" and pertains to the yolk of an egg or ovum. Meckel's diverticulum is a persistence of the vitello-intestinal duct that appears briefly in the embryo and usually disappears.

**Ovum** is Latin for "egg." Synovium means "with egg"; that is, "white of egg."

**Trabs** was a beam in ancient Rome and today its diminutive plural trabeculae means "little beams" or "bars."

**Arytaina** meant a pitcher in ancient Greece and has lent its name to the two arytenoid cartilages in the larynx.

**Ansa** is "handle" in Latin and is used for certain structures that form a loop.

**Zygon** is Greek for "yoke," but could also be used for any of the following: "cross-bar," "pair," "team," "balance," "row," and "line."

**Salpinx** in ancient Greece was a trumpet.

**Trochlea** is "pulley" in Latin.

**Funis** is a rope. Funis is not currently used, but its diminutive funiculus–"little rope"–is applied to bundles of nerve fibers within the white matter of the spinal cord.

**Calix** meant a "cup" in Latin and is derived from the Greek kalyx which could mean a "husk," "shell," "cup," "bud," or "pendant of the ear."

**Falx** was a Roman sickle or scythe.

**The trigeminal nerve** is called the triplet nerve because it divides into three large branches: the ophthalmic nerve, the maxillary nerve, and the mandibular nerve. *Gemini* means "twins" and quadrigemini is "quadruplets."

trigemini (Lat., triplets)

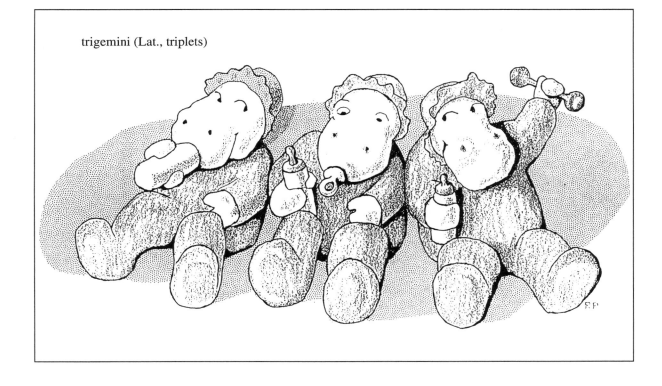

## SECTION 14
## Eyes, Nasal Cavity Level

*Color and label:*

1. Skin of scalp
2. Frontal diploic vein
3. Frontal bone
4. Bone of frontal crest
5. Frontal lobe of brain
6. Galea aponeurotica (epicranial aponeurosis)—extends from frontalis muscle anteriorly to occipitalis muscle posteriorly
7. Loose connective tissue layer of scalp
8. Frontal branch of superficial temporal vein
9. Terminal branch of frontopolar artery (branch of anterior cerebral artery)
10. Frontal sinuses (right and left)
11. Supraorbital nerve
12. Superior ophthalmic vein
13. Superior rectus muscle (tendon)
14. Tendon of superior oblique muscle within trochlea
15. Lacrimal gland
16. Sclera of eye
17. Choroid layer of eye (dark pigmented layer)
18. Crista galli
19. Nasal cavities and left middle nasal concha
20. Maxillary sinus
21. Nasal septum (perpendicular plate of ethmoid above, septal cartilage and vomer below)
22. Levator labii superioris muscle (facial expression)
23. Superior alveolar nerve (left)
24. Anterior nasal spine
25. Maxilla
26. Root and pulp cavity of upper left canine in maxilla
27. Facial artery (above), superior labial artery (below)
28. Buccinator muscle
29. Submandibular ducts opening in sublingual papillae (caruncles)
30. Inferior labial artery
33. Depressor labii inferioris muscle
32. Mentalis muscle
33. Superior alveolar nerves and artery (right)
34. Infraorbital nerve
35. Inferior nasal concha and inferior nasal meatus (beneath and lateral to inferior nasal concha)
36. Middle nasal concha
37. Inferior oblique muscle
38. Ethmoid air cells (sinuses)
39. Nasolacrimal duct
40. Superficial temporal vein and artery (frontal branch)
41. Anterior temporal diploic veins
42. Tendon of levator palpebrae superioris muscle
43. Orbital fat
44. Terminal branch of sphenopalatine artery in incisive canal

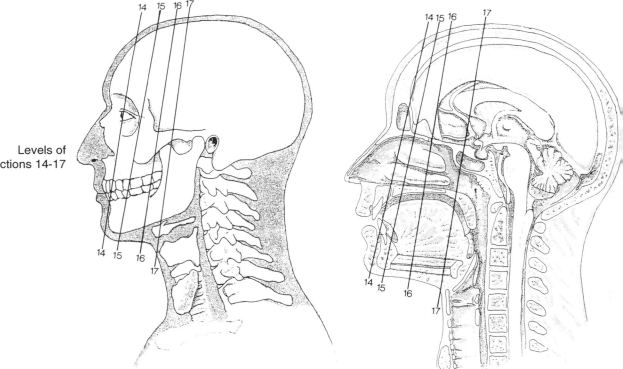

Levels of
Sections 14-17

viewed from
the front

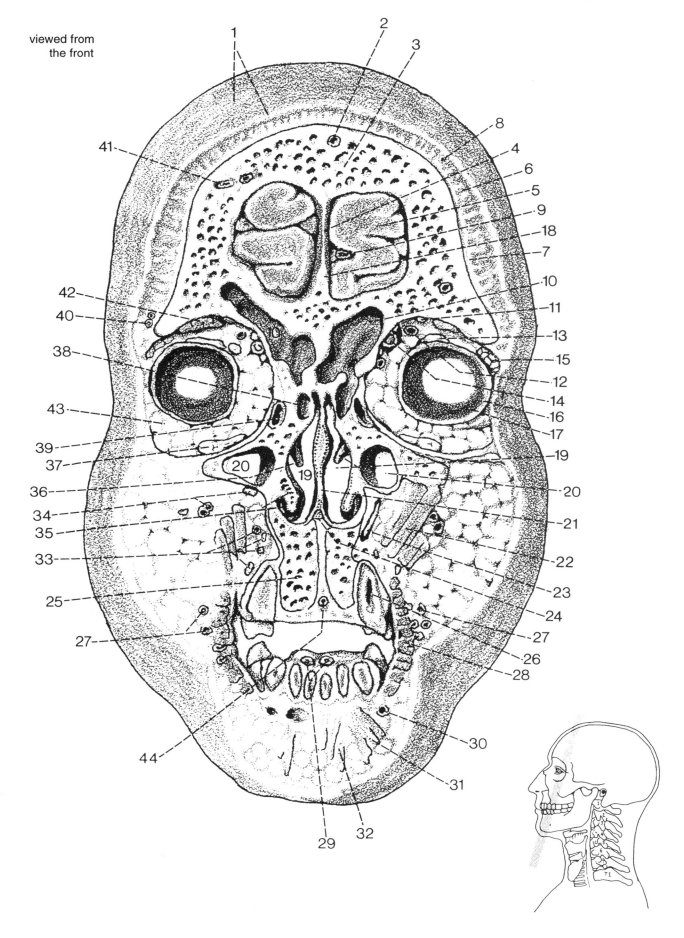

## SECTION 15
## Eye Muscles, Sinuses Level

*Color and label:*

1. Falx cerebri
2. Superior sagittal sinus
3. Dura mater
4. Diploic veins
5. Superior frontal gyrus
6. Middle frontal gyrus
7. Anterior temporal diploic vein
8. Inferior frontal gyrus
9. Gyrus rectus (straight gyrus)
10. Superficial temporal artery (frontal branch)
11. Supraorbital nerve and artery
12. Superficial temporal vein (frontal branch)
13. Lacrimal nerve
14. Superior rectus and levator palpebrae muscles
15. Superior ophthalmic vein and ophthalmic artery,
16. Fundus of eye (back portion)—retina (inner gray) and choroid layer (dark pigmented middle coat)
17. Sclera of eye (outer white fibrous coat of eyeball)
18. Superior oblique muscle (above), medial rectus muscle (below)
19. Inferior rectus muscle and inferior division of oculomotor nerve
20. Infraorbital nerve and infraorbital artery
21. Ethmoid bone (orbital plate—lamina papyracea)
22. Ethmoid air cells (sinuses)
23. Middle nasal concha and middle nasal meatus (space)
24. Maxillary sinus
25. Nasal septum (perpindicular plate of ethmoid bone above and vomer below)
26. Greater palatine artery and nerve
27. Facial nerve—buccal branches
28. Hard palate (maxillary portion) and glands in mucosa of hard palate
29. Buccinator muscle
30. Buccal branch of facial nerve
31. Facial artery
32. Labial arteries and mandibular branches of facial nerve
33. Platysma muscle
34. Submandibular duct and sublingual gland
35. Inferior alveolar nerve in mandible
36. Genioglossus muscle
37. Mandible
38. Submental veins
39. Sublingual vein (in sublingual gland) and inferior alveolar nerve in mandibular canal
40. Tongue
41. Oral cavity
42. Root of tooth in mandible
43. Facial artery and buccal branches of facial nerve
44. Root of tooth in maxilla
45. Facial vein and buccal branches of facial nerve
46. Inferior nasal concha (turbinate) and inferior nasal meatus (space)
47. Nasal cavity
48. Infraorbital vein, nerve, and artery
49. Inferior rectus (extraocular) muscle
50. Orbital fat
51. Lateral rectus (extraocular) muscle
52. Zygomatic bone
53. Medial rectus (extraocular) muscle
54. Optic nerve
55. Lacrimal gland
56. Superior oblique muscle (medial), superior rectus muscle, levator palpebrae muscle (directly above superior rectus)
57. Crista galli (in midline) and cribriform plate (both part of ethmoid bone)
58. Medial orbitofrontal artery (branch of anterior cerebral artery)
59. Frontopolar artery (branch of anterior cerebral artery)
60. Frontal bone
61. Branches of ascending frontal artery (candelabra artery) of middle cerebral artery
62. Cerebral cortex (gray matter)—contains 6 layers of nerve cell bodies
63. White matter (largely myelinated axons)

viewed from
the front

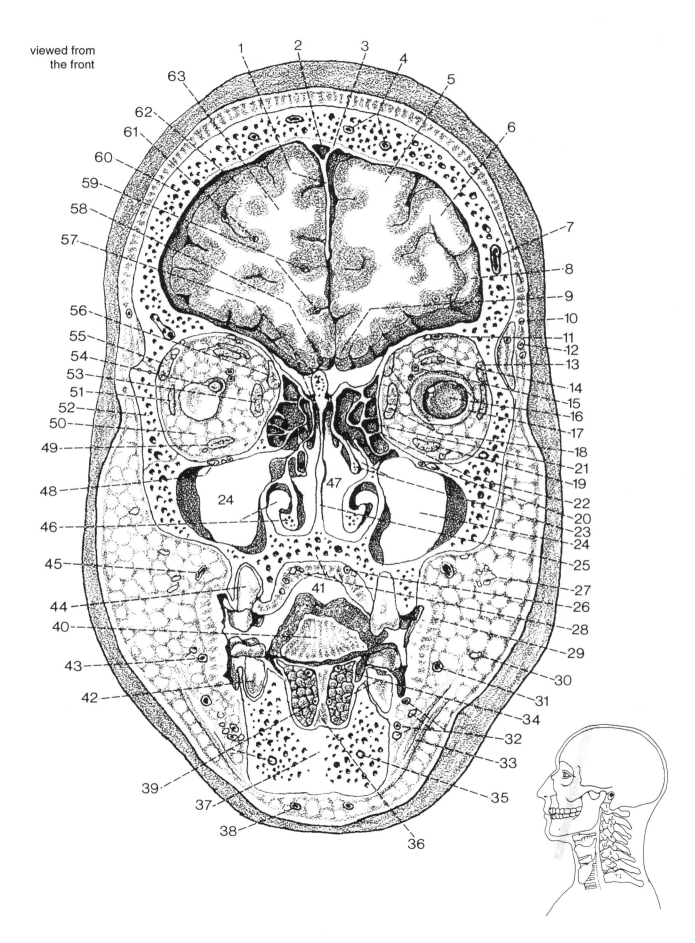

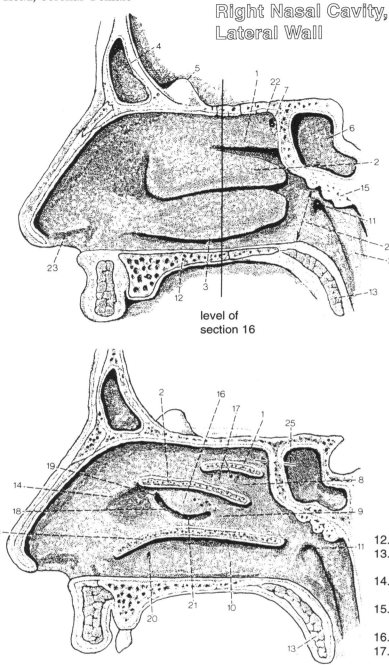

**Right Nasal Cavity, Lateral Wall**

level of section 16

**SECTION 16**
**Maxillary Sinuses Level**

*Color and label (at right):*

1. Superior nasal concha (cut in lower figure)
2. Middle nasal concha (cut in lower figure)
3. Inferior nasal concha (cut in lower figure)
4. Frontal sinus
5. Crista galli
6. Sphenoidal sinus
7. Opening of sphenoidal sinus
8. Superior nasal meatus
9. Middle nasal meatus
10. Inferior nasal meatus
11. Opening of auditory (eustachian) tube
12. Hard palate
13. Soft palate
14. Agger (Lat., mound) nasi
15. Pharyngeal tonsil (called adenoids when inflamed)
16. Ethmoidal bulla (Lat., swelling)
17. Openings of ethmoidal air cells
18. Hiatus semilunaris
19. Opening of frontal sinus into hiatus semilunaris
20. Opening of nasolacrimal duct into inferior nasal meatus
21. Opening of maxillary sinus into hiatus semilunaris
22. Sphenoethmoidal recess
23. Nasal vestibule
24. Choana (posterior opening of nasal cavity into nasal pharynx)
25. Probe in opening of sphenoidal sinus
26. Nasal pharynx (nasopharynx)

*Color and label (at right):*

1. Superior sagittal sinus
2. Longitudinal cerebral fissure (space between cerebral hemispheres)
3. Callosomarginal artery (branch of anterior cerebral artery)
4. Superior frontal gyrus
5. Anterior cerebral arteries curving upwards in front genu of corpus callosum (become pericallosal arteries)
6. Frontal bone
7. Frontal tributary of superficial temporal vein
8. Middle frontal gyrus
9. Anterior temporal diploic vein
10. Straight gyrus (gyrus rectus) of frontal lobe
11. Orbital gyrus of frontal lobe
12. Inferior frontal gyrus
13. Lateral orbitofrontal artery (branch of middle cerebral artery)
14. Levator palpebrae superioris muscle, frontal nerve, superior rectus muscle
15. Superior ophthalmic vein (medial), lacrimal nerve (lateral)
16. Superficial temporal vein and artery
17. Optic nerve in optic canal, ophthalmic artery (immediately above the nerve), lateral rectus muscle
18. Superior oblique muscle (above), medial rectus muscle (immediately below)
19. Inferior rectus muscle, infraorbital nerve (in infraorbital groove in floor of orbit)
20. Temporalis muscle
21. Zygomatic arch
22. Ethmoid air cells (sinuses)
23. Left maxillary sinus
24. Masseter muscle (a small portion)
25. Inferior nasal concha (turbinate), inferior nasal meatus
26. Parotid duct, buccal branches of facial nerve
27. Greater palatine artery and nerve (branch of maxillary nerve in mucosa of hard palate)
28. Molar teeth in maxilla (above) and mandible (below)
29. Buccinator muscle, facial vein
30. Septum of tongue, dorsal lingual vein
31. Facial artery, mandibular branches of facial nerve

*Continued...*

32. Inferior alveolar nerve, vein, and artery in mandibular canal
33. Submandibular duct immediately above lingual nerve
34. Genioglossus muscle, deep lingual vein
35. Hypoglossal nerve (above), sublingual branch of lingual artery (below)
36. Mylohyoid muscle, mylohyoid nerve
37. Anterior belly of digastric muscle (left)
38. Sublingual gland
39. Submental vein
40. Geniohyoid muscles (right and left)
41. Genioglossus muscle (right side)
42. Anterior belly of right digastric muscle
43. Hypoglossal nerve medial to lingual artery
44. Sublingual gland
45. Inferior alveolar nerve, vein, artery in mandibular canal
46. Facial artery and mandibular branch(es) of facial nerve
47. Submandibular duct (lingual nerve just below)
48. Mandible
49. Buccinator muscle, facial vein
50. Lingual mucosa on dorsum of tongue
51. Oral cavity
52. Parotid duct (buccal branches of facial nerve)
53. Glands of hard palate
54. Right maxillary sinus
55. Right nasal cavity
56. Left nasal cavity
57. Zygomatic arch
58. Middle nasal concha, middle nasal meatus
59. Lateral rectus muscle
60. Lacrimal nerve (lateral), frontal nerve (medial)
61. Greater wing of shenoid bone
62. Orbital plate of frontal bone
63. Medial orbitofrontal artery and olfactory tract
64. Anterior cerebral arteries
65. Anterior temporal diploic vein
66. Frontal lobe of cerebral hemisphere (white matter)
67. Cingulate gyrus
68. Galea aponeurotica or epicranial aponeurosis
69. Cingulate sulcus
70. Falx cerebri
71. Lingual artery
72. Buccal fat pad

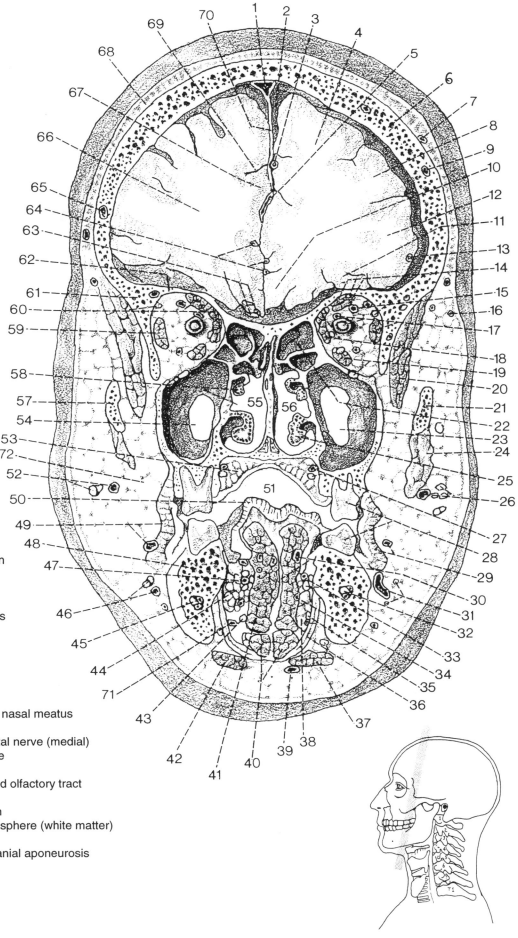

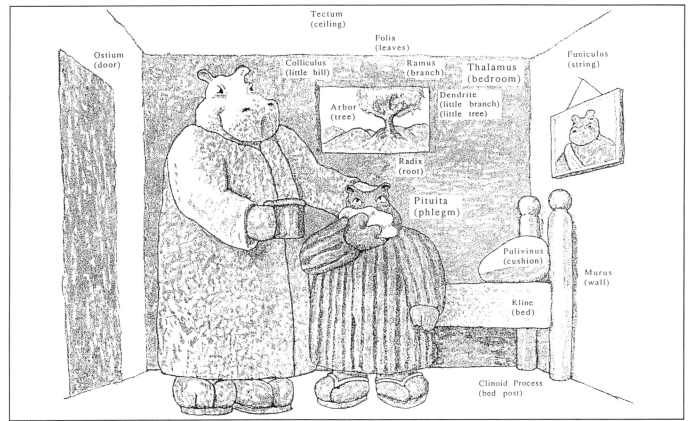

Tectum (ceiling)

Folia (leaves)

Ostium (door)

Colliculus (little hill)

Ramus (branch)

Thalamus (bedroom)

Funiculus (string)

Dendrite (little branch) (little tree)

Arbor (tree)

Radix (root)

Pituita (phlegm)

Pulivinus (cushion)

Murus (wall)

Kline (bed)

Clinoid Process (bed post)

## SECTION 17
## Sphenoid Sinuses Level

*Color and label (at right):*

1. Superior sagittal sinus
2. Subarachnoid space (contains cerebrospinal fluid, traversed by arachnoid trabeculae)—usually is obliterated after death by arachnoid mater separating from dura mater and collapsing on pia mater
3. Falx cerebri
4. Callosomarginal artery (branch of anterior cerebral)
5. Pericallosal artery (continuation of anterior cerebral artery)
6. Anterior temporal diploic vein
7. Corpus callosum (genu)
8. Lateral ventricle (left)
9. Caudate nucleus (head) abutting lateral ventricle
10. Parietal branch of middle cerebral artery
11. Lateral (Sylvian) fissure
12. Superficial middle cerebral vein
13. Middle cerebral artery
14. Anterior temporal artery (off posterior cerebral artery)
15. Deep temporal arterial branch (off maxillary artery), deep temporal nerve (off motor root of V3), and vein in temporalis muscle
16. Zygomatic arch
17. Greater and lesser palatine nerves descending within palatine canal(s) from pterygopalatine fossa to oral cavity
18. Parotid duct, buccal branch of facial nerve
19. Masseter muscle
20. Facial vein
21. Inferior alveolar nerve, artery, and vein inside mandibular canal

22. Left submandibular duct (superior) and lingual nerve (inferior) within sublingual gland
23. Submental artery and vein, submandibular gland
24. Geniohyoid muscles (right and left), septum of tongue
25. Digastric muscle
26. Mylohyoid muscle
27. Hypoglossal nerve (inferior), lingual artery (superior)
28. Right submandibular duct (superior) and lingual nerve (inferior) within sublingual gland
29. Facial artery
30. Inferior alveolar nerve, artery, and vein inside mandibular canal
31. Facial vein
32. Palatine glands in mucosa of hard palate, greater palatine nerve
33. Inferior alveolar artery, vein, and nerve headed toward mandibular foramen
34. Parotid duct, buccal branches of facial nerve, transverse facial artery
35. Coronoid process of mandible, masseter muscle
36. Inferior nasal concha (turbinate), nasal septum (vomer)
37. Temporalis muscle and maxillary artery in infratemporal fossa
38. Zygomatic arch and tendon of temporalis muscle
39. Maxillary nerve
40. Optic nerve and ophthalmic artery within optic canal
41. Superficial temporal artery and vein (frontal branches)
42. Anterior clinoid process
43. Temporal lobe of brain

*Continued...*

viewed from
the front

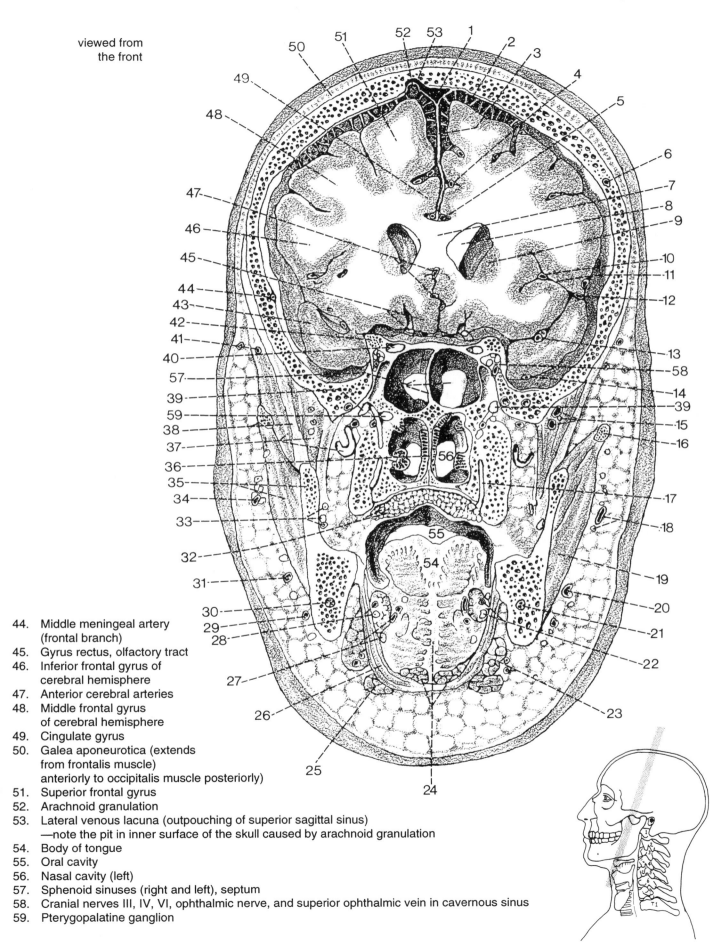

44. Middle meningeal artery
    (frontal branch)
45. Gyrus rectus, olfactory tract
46. Inferior frontal gyrus of
    cerebral hemisphere
47. Anterior cerebral arteries
48. Middle frontal gyrus
    of cerebral hemisphere
49. Cingulate gyrus
50. Galea aponeurotica (extends
    from frontalis muscle)
    anteriorly to occipitalis muscle posteriorly)
51. Superior frontal gyrus
52. Arachnoid granulation
53. Lateral venous lacuna (outpouching of superior sagittal sinus)
    —note the pit in inner surface of the skull caused by arachnoid granulation
54. Body of tongue
55. Oral cavity
56. Nasal cavity (left)
57. Sphenoid sinuses (right and left), septum
58. Cranial nerves III, IV, VI, ophthalmic nerve, and superior ophthalmic vein in cavernous sinus
59. Pterygopalatine ganglion

## SECTION 18
## Optic Chiasm Level

*Color and label:*

1. Sagittal suture
2. Falx cerebri
3. Pericallosal artery (continuation of anterior cerebral artery)
4. Corpus callosum
5. Septum pellucidum (the two septa appear to be fused together)
6. Lateral ventricle (left)
7. Squamosal suture (between temporal and parietal bones)
8. Lateral fissure (of Sylvius)
9. Middle cerebral artery
10. Internal carotid artery (cut at 10 and again at 12, here as part of circle of Willis)
11. Oculomotor nerve (in lateral wall of cavernous sinus)
12. Internal carotid artery (here coursing forward within cavernous sinus)
13. Abducens nerve (above) and maxillary nerve (below)
14. Middle meningeal artery and vein (doubled)
15. Zygomatic process of temporal bone
16. Lateral pterygoid muscle, nerve to lateral pterygoid (from the motor portion of the trigeminal nerve), branches of maxillary artery
17. Masseter muscle
18. Buccal nerve (sensory branch of mandibular nerve)
19. Parotid duct (buccal branch of facial nerve)
20. Inferior alveolar nerve and artery in mandibular canal
21. Medial pterygoid muscle
22. Nerve to mylohyoid
23. Lingual nerve (lateral), styloglossus muscle (medial)
24. Facial vein with mandibular branch of facial nerve
25. Facial artery
26. Submandibular duct
27. Submandibular gland
28. Hypoglossal nerve (lateral) and lingual artery (medial), separated by hyoglossus muscle

29. Infrahyoid muscles (strap muscles of the neck)
30. Cricothyroid muscle
31. Thyroid cartilage
32. Sublingual glands (right and left)
33. Hyoid bone
34. Mylohyoid muscle
35. Lingual artery (medial), submandibular gland (lateral)
36. Hyoglossus muscle
37. Lingual septum, intrinsic tongue muscles
38. Lingual nerve (lateral), styloglossus muscle (medial)
39. Uvula (in midline) and underside of soft palate
40. Mylohyoid nerve (also supplies anterior belly of diagastric muscle)
41. Inferior alveolar artery, vein, and nerve in mandible
42. Tensor veli palatini muscle, lesser palatine nerve and vessels
43. Levator veli palatini muscle
44. Parotid duct, buccal branch of facial nerve
45. Posterior wall of nasopharynx (site of pharyngeal tonsil) viewed through posterior aperature of nasal cavity
46. Auditory (eustachian) tube—cartilaginous part
47. Zygomatic arch (zygomatic process of temporal bone)
48. Sphenoidal sinus and septum
49. Pituitary gland (hypophysis) in sella turcica, infundibulum (pituitary stalk)
50. Optic chiasm
51. Squamosal suture
52. Anterior cerebral arteries
53. Superior sagittal sinus
54. Soft palate (sectioned)
55. Middle cerebral artery (above), anterior clinoid process (below)
56. Middle cerebral artery
57. Medial pterygoid plate
58. Lateral pterygoid plate

Levels of
Sections 18-21

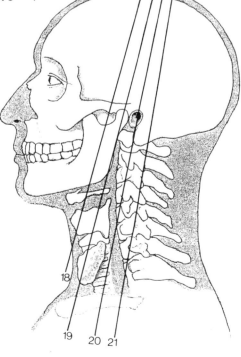

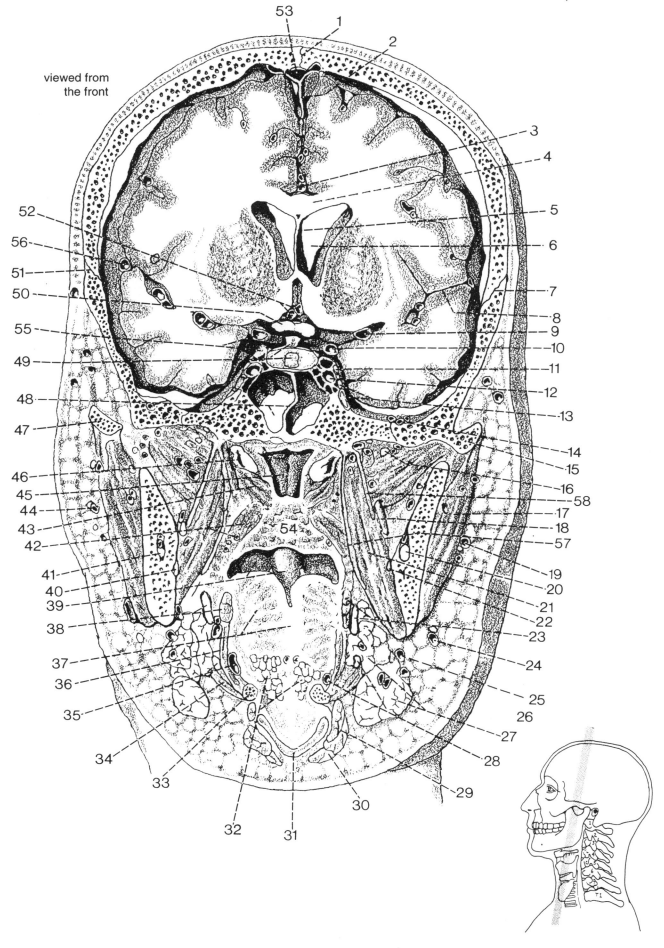

viewed from
the front

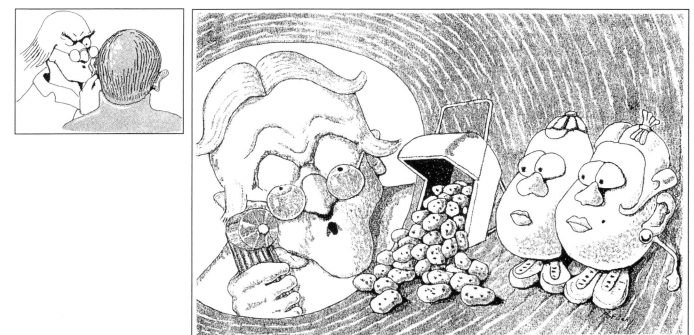

**A physician who specializes in the ears, nose, and throat** is an otorhinolaryngologist (Gr., *ous, otikos*–"ear" + *rhis, rhin*–"nose" + *larynx*–"larynx" + *logos, logy*–"word, study, science") or, simply, an ENT (ear, nose, throat) doctor. This discovery of Mr. and Mrs. Potato Head with their baby carriage of tiny potatoes in the external auditory meatus explains one of the great mysteries of medicine; namely, how potatoes really get in the ears. "Potatoes in the ears" are, of course, actually mothers' threats that "potatoes will grow in your ears" if you don't clean out the ear wax or cerumen. This cartoon won't mean much to you if your mother never chided you about potatoes growing in your ears.

## SECTION 19
## Carotid Canal Level

*Color and label:*

1. Superior sagittal sinus
2. Falx cerebri
3. Cingulate gyrus
4. Corpus callosum
5. Lateral ventricle
6. Septum pellucidum (right and left fused together)
7. Fornix (body)—both right and left
8. Ventricle III
9. Superficial temporal artery
10. Inferior (temporal) horn of lateral ventricle
11. Trigeminal ganglion
12. Internal carotid artery in carotid canal in temporal bone
13. Superficial temporal artery
14. Auriculotemporal nerve (medial) and small part of mandible head (lateral)
15. Maxillary vein
16. Parotid duct
17. Parotid gland
18. Pharyngeal constrictor muscles
19. Hyoid bone
20. Posterior wall of pharynx
21. Arytenoid cartilage
22. Thyroid cartilage
23. Cricoid cartilage
24. Cricothyroid muscle
25. Sternocleidomastoid muscle (clavicular head)
26. Clavicle (left)
27. Sternothyroid and sternohyoid muscles
28. Infraglottic space (below the vocal folds)—back wall is mucosal-lined lamina of the cricoid cartilage
29. Thyroid gland (right lateral lobe)
30. Clavicle (right)
31. Thyro-arytenoid muscle
32. Thyrohyoid muscle
33. Thyrohyoid membrane (white band between thyroid cartilage and hyoid bone)
34. Superior laryngeal nerve (branch of N X)
35. Submandibular gland
36. Hypoglossal nerve (N XII)
37. Intermediate tendon of digastric muscle (connects its two bellies)
38. Stylohyoid muscle
39. Stylopharyngeus muscle and glossopharnngeal nerve (N IX)
40. Styloglossus muscle
41. Anterior tubercle of atlas (C1), longus capitis muscle

*Continued...*

viewed from
the front

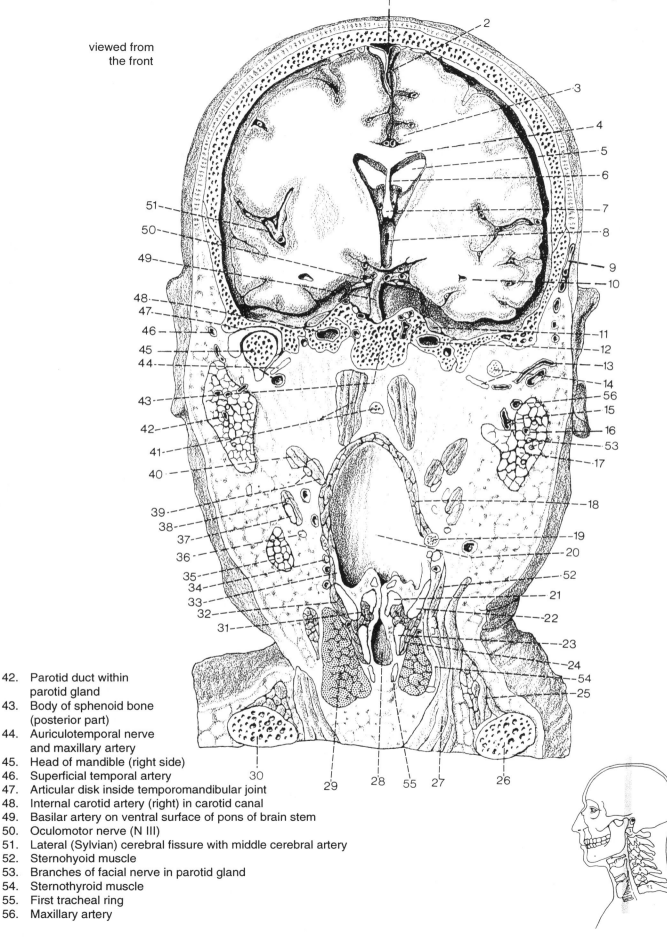

42. Parotid duct within
    parotid gland
43. Body of sphenoid bone
    (posterior part)
44. Auriculotemporal nerve
    and maxillary artery
45. Head of mandible (right side)
46. Superficial temporal artery
47. Articular disk inside temporomandibular joint
48. Internal carotid artery (right) in carotid canal
49. Basilar artery on ventral surface of pons of brain stem
50. Oculomotor nerve (N III)
51. Lateral (Sylvian) cerebral fissure with middle cerebral artery
52. Sternohyoid muscle
53. Branches of facial nerve in parotid gland
54. Sternothyroid muscle
55. First tracheal ring
56. Maxillary artery

**The sella turcica is a bony, saddle-like structure** under the brain and atop the body of the sphenoid bone. The pituitary gland sits snugly within this bony hollow. Four bony projections at its corners, which resemble small bed posts, are called clinoid processes (Gr., *kline*–"bed" + *eidos*–"form").

The Romans rode their horses with no saddles, only a cloth ephipppium tied to the back of the horse. The Arabs and Turks, on the other hand, used elaborate saddles with both front and back supports, and it was these saddles that the ancient anatomists had in mind when they named this bony structure.

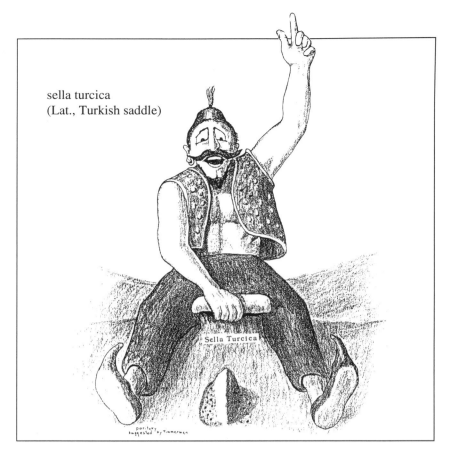

sella turcica
(Lat., Turkish saddle)

## SECTION 20
### Pons, Internal Jugular Vein Level

*Color and label:*

1. Superior sagittal sinus
2. Falx cerebri
3. Cingulate gyrus
4. Corpus callosum
5. Left lateral ventricle
6. Fornix
7. Lateral (Sylvian) fissure
8. Superior temporal gyrus
9. Inferior (temporal) horn of left lateral ventricle
10. Middle temporal gyrus
11. Inferior temporal gyrus
12. Edge of tentorium cerebelli
13. Facial nerve and vestibulocochlear nerve in internal auditory (acoustic) meatus
14. Air cells in temporal bone
15. Vestibule (cavity containing utricle and saccule) of inner ear
16. External auditory meatus (ear canal)
17. Left hypoglossal nerve (N XII) in hypoglossal canal
18. Facial nerve (N VII) descending through facial canal in petrous temporal bone
19. Occipital condyle
20. Facial nerve branches within parotid gland
21. Parotid duct within parotid gland
22. Atlanto-occipital joint (joint between vertebra C1 and occipital condyles at base of skull)
23. Odontoid process (dens) of C2 (axis)
24. Dorsal root ganglion of cervical spinal nerve C2
25. Internal jugular vein (left)—cut in several places
26. Internal carotid artery
27. Maxillary vein
28. Sternocleidomastoid muscle
29. Common carotid artery (left)
30. Thoracic duct
31. Clavicle (left)
32. Subclavian vein
33. Esophagus
34. Lymph glands
35. Thyroid gland
36. Clavicle (right)
37. Internal jugular vein (right)
38. Common carotid artery (right)
39. Sympathetic trunk (right)
40. Vagus nerve (right)
41. Longus colli muscle
42. Cervical vertebra C3
43. Cervical vertebra C2
44. Atlanto-axial joint (joint between cervical vertebrae C1 and C2) and right vagus nerve (N X)
45. Stylohyoid ligament and stylohyoid muscle
46. Internal jugular vein (right)
47. Parotid duct and facial nerve branches in parotid gland
48. Basilar artery on ventral medulla
49. Hypoglossal nerve (right)
50. Facial nerve (right) within facial canal
51. Tympanic cavity (middle ear, lateral) and cochlea (medial)

*Continued...*

viewed from
the front

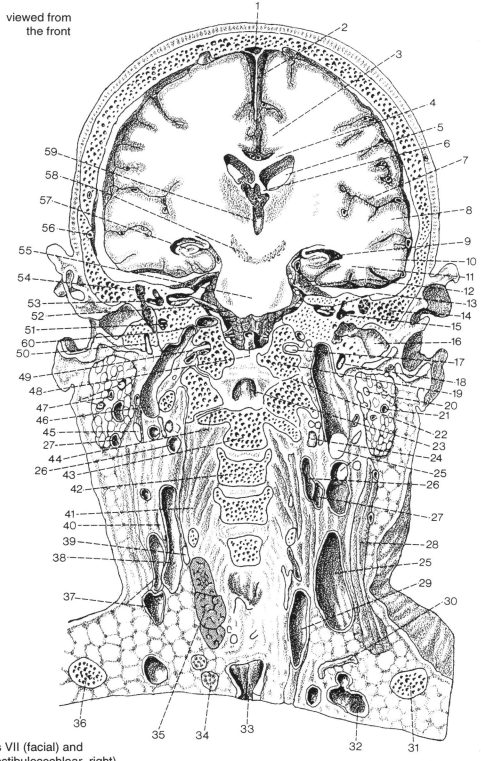

52. Nerves VII (facial) and
    VIII (vestibulocochlear, right)
    entering internal auditory meatus
53. Vestibule of right inner ear
54. Epitympanic recess (upper compartment of middle ear)
55. Pons
56. Middle meningeal artery
57. Hippocampal formation within temporal lobe of brain
58. Substantia nigra of midbrain
59. Ventricle III
60. Jugular foramen

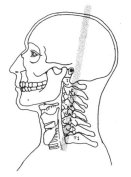

**Latin names for parts of the nervous system**

1. Locus ceruleus—blue place
2. Tectum—roof
3. Vitrum—glass
4. Fenestra—window
5. Lithos (Gr.)—rock
6. Lemniscus—ribbon
7. Brachia conjunctiva—arms that come together
8. Macula—spot
9. Substantia gelatinosa—jelly-like substance
10. Ampulla—flask
11. Genu—knee
12. Peduncle—little foot
13. Operculum—cover or lid
14. Amygdala—almond
15. Putamen—shell
16. Uncus—hook
17. Decussate—to cut in the form of an X

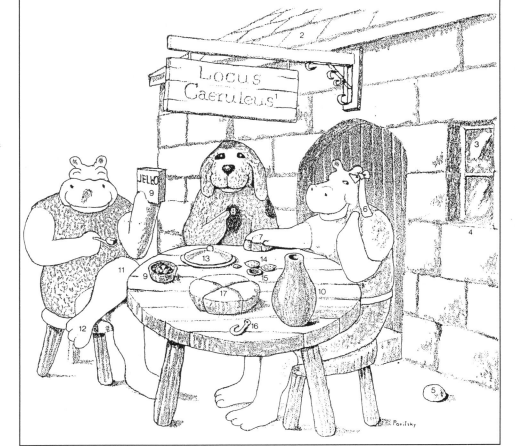

## SECTION 21
## Dens of Axis Level

*Color and label:*

1. Superior sagittal sinus
2. Lateral lacuna (outpouching) of superior sagittal sinus
3. Falx cerebri
4. Diploic vein
5. Cingulate gyrus
6. Pericallosal arteries (continuation of anterior cerebral arteries)
7. Corpus callosum
8. Lateral ventricle
9. Fornix
10. Pineal gland
11. Inferior (temporal) horn of lateral ventricle and choroid plexus
12. Ventricle IV (narrow superior end approaching cerebral aqueduct)
13. Tentorium cerebelli
14. Superior petrosal sinus
15. Cerebellar hemisphere
16. Sigmoid sinus
17. Lesser occipital nerve
18. Mastoid air cells in mastoid process
19. Odontoid process (dens) of cervical vertebra C2
20. Accessory nerve (N XI)
21. Vertebral artery (left)
22. Great auricular nerve (cutaneous branch of cervical plexus)
23. External jugular vein
24. Spinal ganglion (dorsal root ganglion) of spinal nerve C3 in intervetebral foramen
25. Spinal cord (anterior surface)
26. Portion of posterior wall of internal jugular vein
27. Sternocleidomastoid muscle
28. Vertebra C5 body
29. Spinal nerve C6
30. Vertebral artery
31. Scalenus medius muscle
32. Clavicle (left)
33. Subclavian artery
34. First rib
35. Vertebra C6 body
36. Esophagus
37. Vertebra C7 body
38. Vertebral artery (right)
39. Brachial plexus
40. Clavicle (right)
41. Vertebra C5 transverse process
42. Ventral rootlets (right) coalescing into ventral root of spinal nerve C5
43. Vertebra C4 transverse process
44. Denticulate ligament
45. Anterior spinal artery

*Continued...*

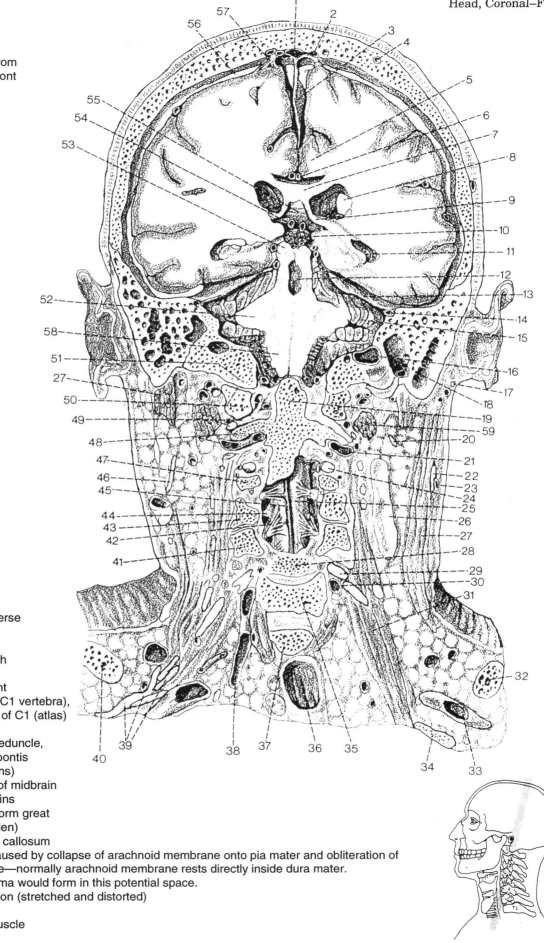

viewed from
the front

46. Accessory nerve
N XI (right)
47. Vertebra C3
transverse process
48. Vertebra C2 transverse
process and right
vertebral artery
49. Spinal nerve C2 with
its dural sheath
50. Atlanto-occipital joint
(between skull and C1 vertebra),
transverse process of C1 (atlas)
51. Occipital condyle
52. Middle cerebellar peduncle,
formerly brachium pontis
(Lat., arm of the pons)
53. Superior colliculus of midbrain
54. Internal cerebral veins
(join posteriorly to form great
cerebral vein of Galen)
55. Splenium of corpus callosum
56. Artifactual space caused by collapse of arachnoid membrane onto pia mater and obliteration of
subarachnoid space—normally arachnoid membrane rests directly inside dura mater.
A subdural hematoma would form in this potential space.
57. Arachnoid granulation (stretched and distorted)
58. Medulla oblongata
59. Anterior scalene muscle

# Thorax/Root of Neck – Male
## Sections 22 to 30

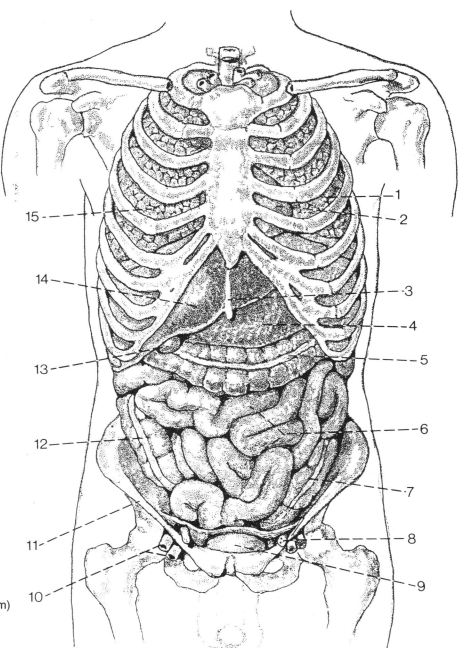

*Color and label:*

1. Left lung
2. Heart
3. Falciform ligament (cut)
4. Stomach
5. Teniae coli on transverse colon
6. Small intestine (jejunum and ileum)
7. Descending colon
8. Spermatic cord
9. Bladder
10. Femoral artery and vein
11. Inguinal ligament
12. Ascending colon
13. Gall bladder
14. Liver (right lobe)
15. Right lung

*after Eycleshymer and Jones*

# Ventricles of the Heart

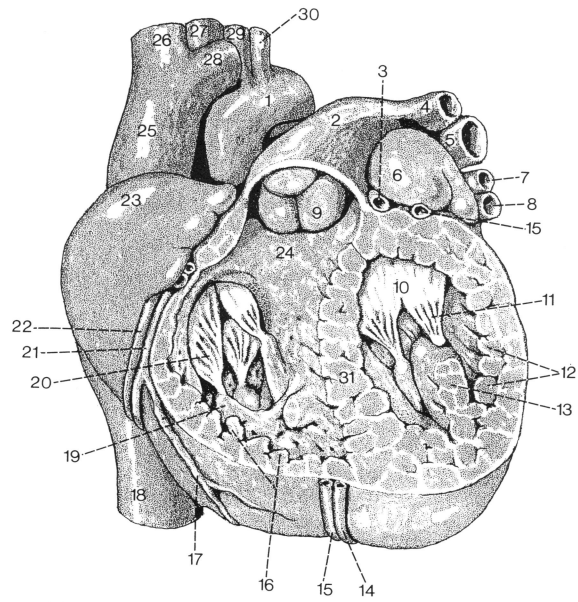

*Color and label\*:*

1. Arch of aorta
2. Pulmonary trunk
3. Anterior interventricular artery (also called left anterior descending)
4. Superior branch of left pulmonary artery
5. Inferior branch of left pulmonary artery
6. Left auricle
7. Left superior pulmonary vein
8. Left inferior pulmonary vein
9. Pulmonary valve
10. Anterior cusp of bicuspid (mitral) valve
11. Chordae tendinae
12. Trabeculae carnae in wall of left ventricle
13. Anterior papillary muscle in left ventricle
14. Anterior interventricular artery
15. Great cardiac vein

16. Trabeculae carnae in wall of right ventricle
17. Right marginal artery
18. Inferior vena cava
19. Papillary muscle
20. Chordae tendineae and cusp of tricuspid valve
21. Right coronary artery
22. Small cardiac vein
23. Right auricle
24. Infundibulum of right ventricle
25. Superior vena cava
26. Right brachiocephalic vein
27. Brachiocephalic artery
28. Left brachiocephalic vein
29. Left common carotid artery
30. Left subclavian artery
31. Interventricular septum

\* Much of anterior wall has been removed to reveal interior of ventricles.

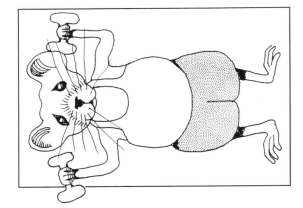

**SECTION 22**
**Thyroid Gland Level**

*Color and label:*

1. Trachea and rima (Lat., crack, fissure, cleft) glottidis–space between vocal cords or folds
2. Sternohyoid muscle
3. Sternothyroid muscle
4. Esophagus and recurrent laryngeal nerve
5. Left common carotid artery and vagus nerve
6. Left internal jugular vein
7. Platysma muscle (external) and omohyoid muscle–inferior belly (internal)
8. Longus colli muscle and vertebral artery
9. Cervical nerve C7 and anterior scalene muscle
10. Left external jugular vein
11. Upper trunk of brachial plexus and middle scalene muscle
12. Left clavicle
13. Top of head of left humerus
14. Spine of scapula
15. Supraspinatus muscle
16. Transverse process of thoracic vertebra T1 articulating with tubercle of first rib
17. Dorsal root ganglion of nerve C8
18. Rhomboid major muscle
19. Superior articular process of thoracic vertebra T1
20. Body of cervical vertebra C7 and intervertebral disk C7-T1
21. Spinal cord (note denticulate ligament on either side)
22. Multifidus and rotatores muscles
23. Semispinalis cervicis muscle
24. Splenius cervicis muscle
25. Longissimus muscle

26. Iliocostalis muscle
27. Spine of right scapula
28. Glenohumeral joint (between glenoid fossa of scapula and head of humerus)
29. Head of humerus
30. Deltoid muscle
31. Infraspinatus muscle
32. Serratus posterior superior muscle
33. Tendon of long head of biceps brachii muscle
34. Suprascapular artery and vein
35. Right clavicle and subclavius muscle
36. Omohyoid muscle (lower belly)
37. Right external jugular vein
38. Posterior scalene muscle
39. Phrenic nerve
40. Right internal jugular vein
41. Sternocleidomastoid muscle
42. Right common carotid artery and vagus nerve
43. Thyroid gland (right lobe)
44. Anterior jugular vein
45. Rhomboid minor muscle
46. Trapezius muscle
47. Labrum of glenoid fossa
48. Levator scapulae muscle
49. Supraspinatus muscle
50. Infraspinatus muscle
51. Teres minor muscle
52. Left scapula (superior angle) and serratus anterior muscle

**The word muscle** originally meant "little mouse" (Lat., *mus*–"mouse"; *musculus*–"little mouse").

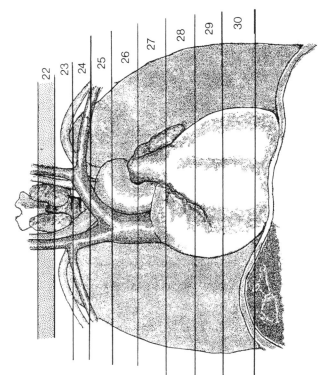

Levels of
Sections 22-30

looking up
from below

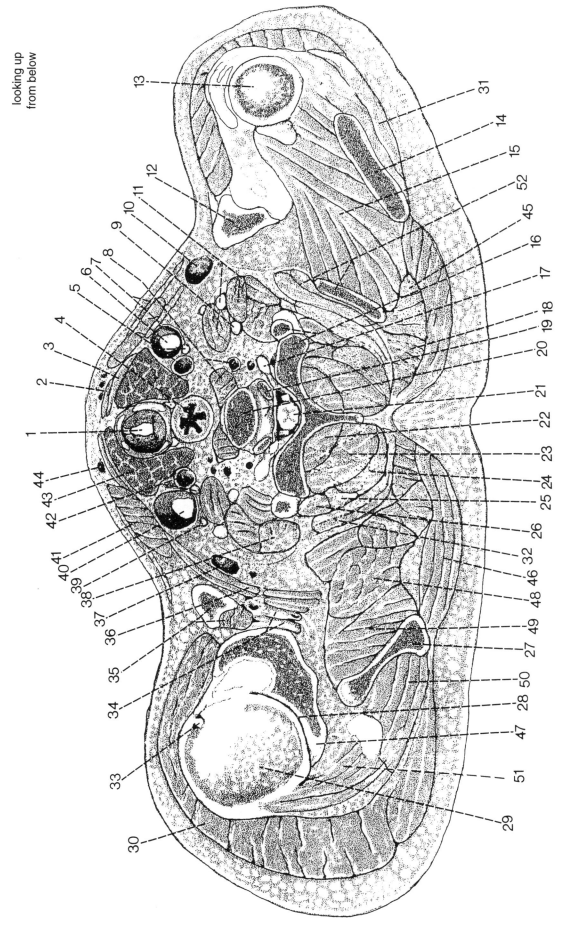

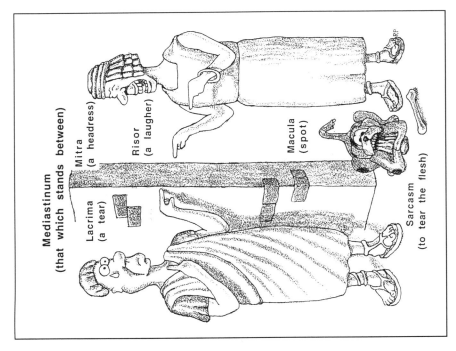

Mediastinum
(that which stands between)

Mitra
(a headress)

Risor
(a laugher)

Lacrima
(a tear)

Macula
(spot)

Sarcasm
(to tear the flesh)

**A sarcastic remark in ancient Rome.** "You're as exciting as a mediastinum," says the woman to the man. She is comparing him to a wall or partition.

**SECTION 23**
**Apex of Lung Level**

*Color and label:*

1. Trachea
2. Esophagus and lymph nodes
3. Anterior jugular vein
4. Left common carotid artery and left vagus nerve
5. Internal jugular vein
6. Left subclavian artery (curving over apex of lung) and internal thoracic artery
7. Vertebral vein
8. External jugular vein
9. Anterior scalene muscle and left phrenic nerve
10. Left subclavian artery
11. Left brachial plexus
12. Coracobrachialis muscle
13. Biceps brachii (short head) muscle
14. Tendon of biceps brachii (long head) in intertubercular groove of humerus
15. Head of humerus and glenohumeral joint
16. Suprascapular artery and vein
17. Infraspinatus muscle
18. Left scapula (note its thinness)
19. Serratus anterior muscle and long thoracic nerve (nerve to serratus anterior)
20. Apex of left lung
21. Serratus posterior superior muscle
22. Spinal cord and superior articular process of thoracic vertebra T2
23. Iliocostalis muscle
24. Longissimus cervicis muscle
25. Longissimus capitis muscle
26. Splenius cervicis muscle
27. Multifidus and semispinalis capitis muscles
28. Spinous process of thoracic vertebra T2
29. Body and inferior articular process of thoracic vertebra T1

30. Transverse process of vertebra T2
31. Rhomboideus major muscle
32. Rib 2 (tubercle)
33. Apex of right lung
34. Rib 1
35. Rib 2
36. Subscapularis muscle
37. Deltoid muscle
38. Right humerus
39. Tendon of long head of biceps brachii muscle
40. Biceps brachii short head and coracobrachialis muscle
41. Cephalic vein
42. Pectoralis major (superficial) and pectoralis minor (deep) muscles
43. Right subclavian artery and lymph node
44. Scalenus anterior muscle
45. Right clavicle and subclavius muscle
46. Platysma muscle
47. Internal jugular vein combining with external jugular vein
48. Right subclavian artery
49. Tendon of sternocleidomastoid muscle (sternal head)
50. Right common carotid artery
51. Sternohyoid muscle (anterior) and sternothyroid muscle (posterior)
52. Right scapula
53. Right brachial plexus
54. Axilla
55. Superior mediastinum
56. Teres major muscle

looking up
from below

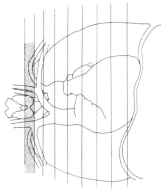

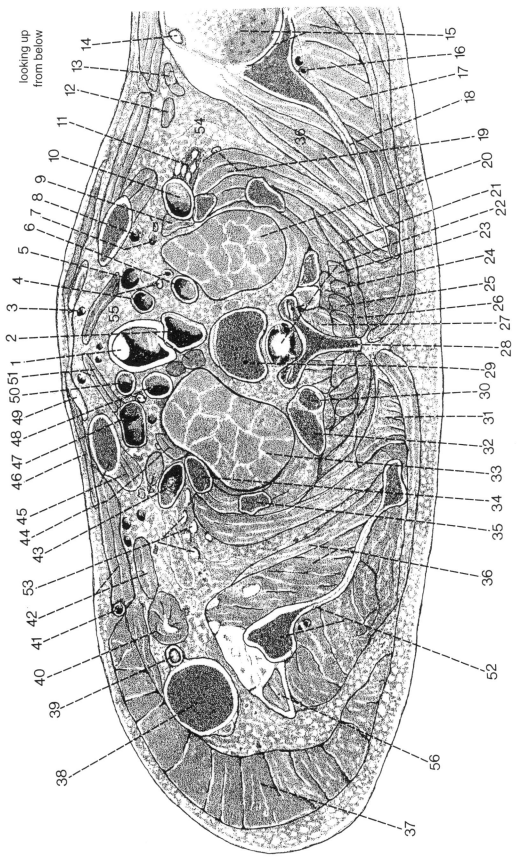

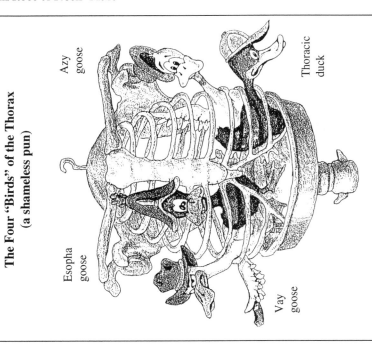

## The Four "Birds" of the Thorax
(a shameless pun)

Azy
goose

Esopha
goose

Thoracic
duck

Vay
goose

**Another shameless play upon words.** The "Esopha goose" represents the esophagus. The "Azy goose" represents the azygos vein. The "Vay goose" represents the vagus nerve. The "Thoracic duck" represents the thoracic duct (the largest lymph vessel in the body). Wayne Timmerman, one of my medical illustration students, drew this cartoon.

## SECTION 24
## Manubrium Level

*Color and label:*

1. Manubrium of sternum
2. Trachea (note C-shaped cartilage in wall)
3. Esophagus
4. Right brachiocephalic vein
5. Brachiocephalic artery
6. Left common carotid artery
7. Left brachiocephalic vein
8. Left subclavian artery
9. Humerus
10. Clavicle, forming sternoclavicular joint with manubrium
11. Internal thoracic artery
12. Left phrenic nerve (more ventral) and left vagus nerve (next to subclavian artery #8)
13. Body of thoracic vertebra T3
14. Left lung upper lobe
15. Left axillary vein
16. Left axillary artery (continuation of left subclavian artery)
17. Coracobrachialis muscle and short head of biceps brachii muscle
18. Tendon of long head of biceps brachii muscle
19. Third rib
20. Long head of triceps brachii muscle
21. Teres minor muscle
22. Infraspinatus muscle
23. Left scapula (note its thinness)
24. Iliocostalis muscle (part of erector spinae muscle)
25. Rhomboideus major muscle
26. Trapezius muscle
27. Longissimus muscle (part of erector spinae muscle)
28. Multifidus and semispinalis muscles
29. Spinal cord, internal vertebral venous plexus
30. Rib 4 articulating with body of vertebra T3 and transverse process of T4
31. Upper lobe of right lung
32. Serratus anterior muscle
33. Subscapularis muscle
34. Right scapula
35. Radial nerve
36. Teres major muscle
37. Axillary nerve
38. Tendon of latissimus dorsi muscle
39. Long head of triceps brachii muscle
40. Lateral head of triceps brachii
41. Deltoid muscle
42. Tendon of long head of biceps brachii
43. Cephalic vein
44. Musculocutaneous nerve
45. Right axillary artery
46. Median nerve
47. Ulnar nerve
48. Right axillary vein
49. Pectoralis major muscle
50. Pectoralis minor muscle
51. Right highest intercostal vein
52. First rib
53. Right vagus nerve
54. Right phrenic nerve, internal thoracic artery
55. Remnants of thymus gland
56. Transverse process of T4
57. Thoracic duct
58. Sympathetic trunk
59. Superior mediastinum

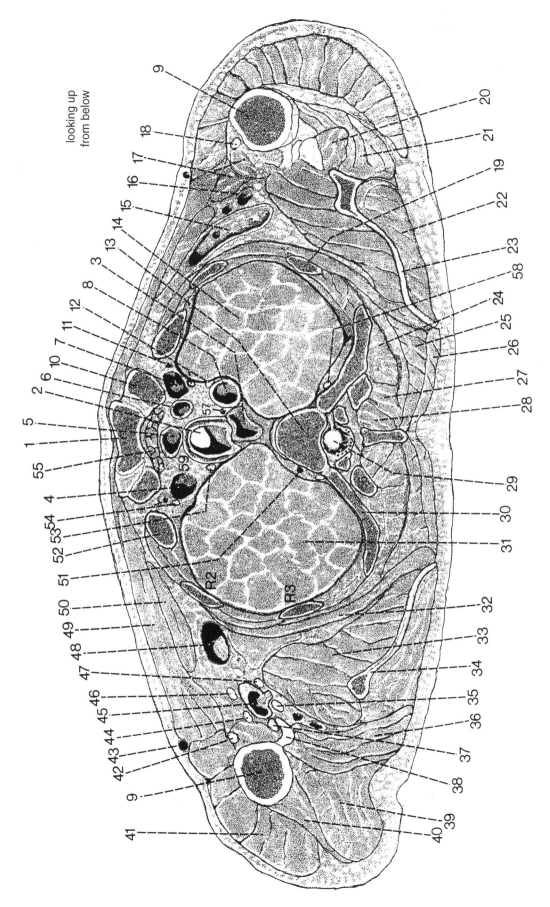

looking up
from below

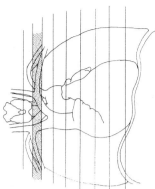

## Heart Exterior

**SECTION 25**
**Aortic Arch Level**

*Color and label (below):*

1. Superior vena cava
2. Trachea
3. Manubrium
4. Brachiocephalic artery
5. Left common carotid artery
6. Internal thoracic artery and vein
7. Arch of the aorta
8. Left subclavian artery
9. Esophagus and left recurrent laryngeal nerve
10. Left lung upper lobe
11. Tendon of long head of left biceps brachii muscle
12. Left scapula
13. Serratus anterior muscle
14. Intercostal muscles
15. Rib 4
16. Lower lobe of left lung
17. Fifth rib (articulating with thoracic vertebra T5)
18. Transverse process of vertebra T5
19. Anterior longitudinal ligament
20. Spinal cord
21. Sympathetic trunk
22. Right highest intercostal vein
23. Trapezius muscle
24. Rhomboideus major muscle
25. Infraspinatus muscle
26. Subscapularis muscle
27. Right scapula
28. Teres minor muscle
29. Circumflex scapular artery and vein
30. Teres major muscle
31. Tendon of latissimus dorsi muscle
32. Nerves of arm from brachial plexus
33. Long head of triceps brachii muscle
34. Lateral head of triceps brachii
35. Deltoid muscle
36. Axillary artery
37. Tendon of long head of right biceps brachii muscle
38. Coracobrachialis (with musculocutaneous nerve) and short head of biceps brachii muscle

*Continued...*

*Color these veins violet (at left):*

1. Right brachiocephalic vein
2. Left brachiocephalic vein
3. Superior vena cava
4. Inferior vena cava
5. Right internal thoracic vein
6. Left internal thoracic vein
7. Right pericardiacophrenic vein
8. Left pericardiacophrenic vein
9. Anterior cardiac veins
10. Great cardiac vein
11. Pulmonary trunk

*Color these arteries red (at left):*

12. Ascending aorta
13. Brachiocephalic artery
14. Right internal thoracic artery
15. Right pericardiacophrenic artery
16. Right common carotid artery
17. Left subclavian artery
18. Left internal thoracic artery
19. Left pericardiacophrenic artery
20. Right coronary artery
21. Marginal branch
22. Anterior interventricular artery (branch of left coronary artery)
23. Cut edge of pericardium
24. Cut edge of pleura

*Color these nerves yellow (at left):*

25. Right phrenic nerve
26. Left phrenic nerve
27. Left vagus nerve
28. Recurrent laryngeal nerve

*Also...*

29. Ligamentum arteriosum
30. Right auricle
31. Left auricle
32. Root of left lung
33. Right ventricle
34. Left ventricle

coronary vessels lie under fat

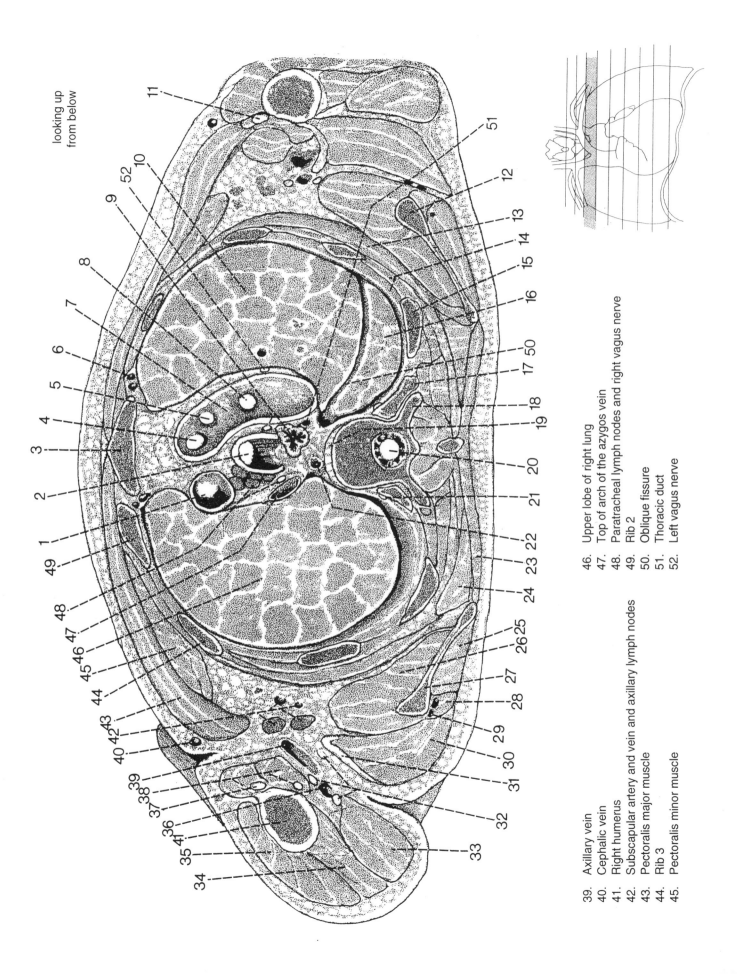

looking up
from below

39. Axillary vein
40. Cephalic vein
41. Right humerus
42. Subscapular artery and vein and axillary lymph nodes
43. Pectoralis major muscle
44. Rib 3
45. Pectoralis minor muscle

46. Upper lobe of right lung
47. Top of arch of the azygos vein
48. Paratracheal lymph nodes and right vagus nerve
49. Rib 2
50. Oblique fissure
51. Thoracic duct
52. Left vagus nerve

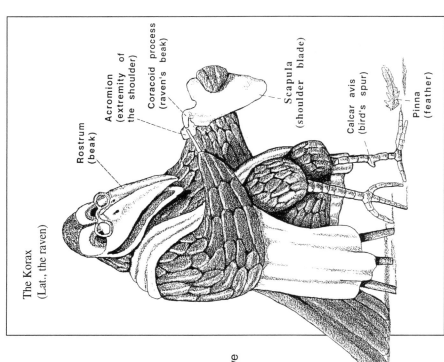

The Korax
(Lat., the raven)

Rostrum
(beak)

Acromion
(extremity of
the shoulder)

Coracoid process
(raven's beak)

Scapula
(shoulder blade)

Calcar avis
(bird's spur)

Pinna
(feather)

**SECTION 26**
**Bifurcation of Pulmonary Trunk Level**

*Color and label:*

1. Remnant of thymus gland and prepericardial fat
2. Sternum (body)
3. Ascending aorta
4. Internal thoracic vein and artery
5. Pulmonary trunk, bifurcation into right and left pulmonary arteries
6. Left main bronchus (note cartilage in walls)
7. Upper lobe of left lung
8. Left phrenic nerve with pericardiacophrenic artery and vein (all three lie sandwiched between pericardial sac and mediastinal pleura)
9. Short head of biceps brachii muscle
10. Long head of biceps brachii and tendon
11. Coracobrachialis muscle
12. Humerus of left arm
13. Deltoid muscle
14. Tendon of latissimus dorsi muscle
15. Lateral head of triceps brachii muscle
16. Long head of triceps brachii
17. Radial nerve
18. Brachial artery
19. Basilic vein
20. Ulnar nerve
21. Median nerve
22. Left scapula
23. Subscapularis muscle
24. Serratus anterior muscle
25. Lower lobe of left lung
26. Left pulmonary artery
27. Semispinalis muscle
28. Descending aorta
29. Head of sixth rib
30. Body of sixth thoracic vertebra and sympathetic trunk
31. Spinous process of vertebra T5
32. Spinal cord
33. Esophagus, azygos vein, and right vagus nerve
34. Trapezius muscle
35. Right main bronchus
36. Right pulmonary artery
37. Lower lobe of right lung
38. Right scapula (inferior angle)
39. Teres major muscle
40. Oblique fissure of right lung
41. Pectoralis major muscle
42. Upper lobe of right lung
43. Pectoralis minor muscle
44. Superior vena cava
45. Cartilage forming keel-like carina at bifurcation of trachea
46. Left vagus nerve

looking up
from below

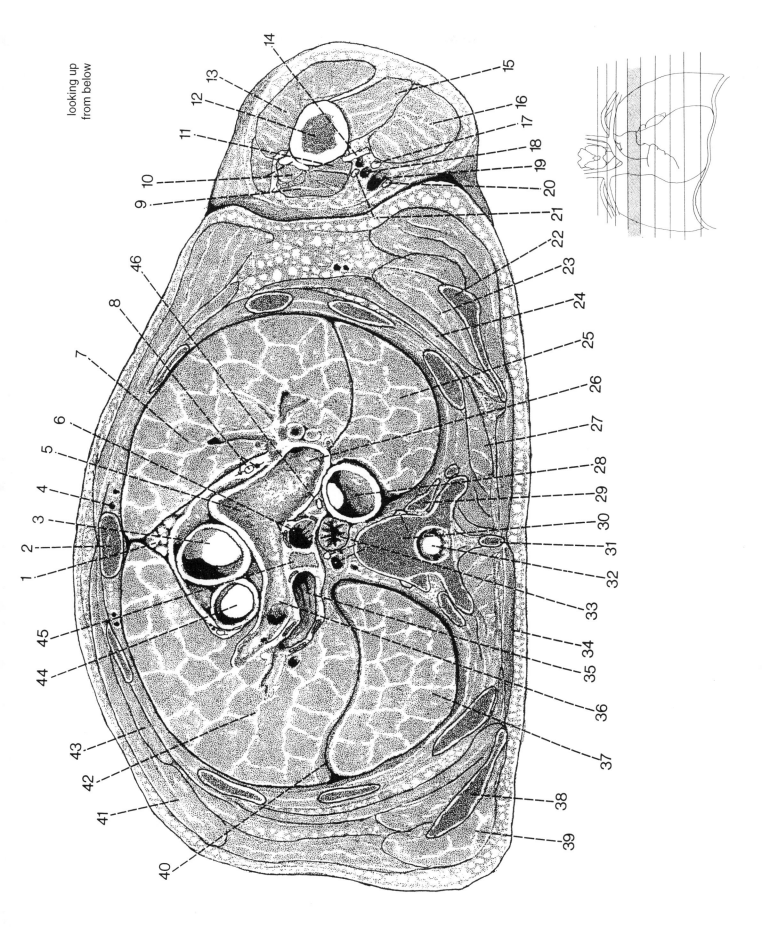

14
13
12
11
15
16
17
18
19
20
21
22
23
24
25
26
27
28
29
30
31
32
33
34
35
36
37
38
39
40
41
42
43
44
45
46
8
7
6
5
4
3
2
1
9
10

# SECTION 27
## Pulmonary Valve Level

*Color and label (below):*

1. Sternum (body)
2. Pulmonary valve seen through infundibulum of right ventricle
3. Left phrenic nerve with pericardiacophrenic artery and vein
4. Superior left pulmonary vein leading into left atrium
5. Left inferior lobar bronchus surrounded with bronchial cartilage
6. Superior lobe of left lung
7. Intercostal muscles
8. Lymph nodes
9. Inferior lobe of left lung
10. Serratus anterior muscle
11. Latissimus dorsi muscle
12. Teres major muscle
13. Subscapularis muscle
14. Scapula (inferior angle)
15. Infraspinatus muscle
16. Esophagus (surrounded by anterior and posterior esophageal plexuses formed by left and right vagus nerves)
17. Rhomboideus major muscle
18. Trapezius muscle
19. Aorta (descending thoracic)
20. Sympathetic trunk
21. Azygos vein
22. Spinous process of thoracic vertebra T6
23. Spinal cord
24. Multifidus (deep) and semispinalis (more superficial) back muscles
25. Body of thoracic vertebra T7
26. Right inferior lobar bronchus with cartilage in its wall
27. Pleural space or cavity, bounded externally by parietal pleura on inside of chest wall and internally by visceral pleura on surface of lung*
28. Right pulmonary artery dividing into lobar branches
29. Inferior angle of right scapula

*Continued...*

*Color and label (at left)\*:*

1. Right coronary artery and branches
2. Main atrial branch, or artery of sinoatrial node
3. Sinoatrial nodal artery (arises from right coronary artery in 55% of hearts examined; from circumflex branch of left coronary artery in 45%)
4. Right conus artery
5. Right anterior ventricular rami
6. Right marginal artery (reaches apex of heart in 93% of hearts examined)
7. Right posterior ventricular rami
8. Posterior interventricular artery
9. Atrioventricular nodal artery (supplies AV node)
10. Anterior atrial rami
11. Left coronary artery and branches
12. Circumflex artery
13. Anterior interventricular artery, or left anterior descending artery
14. Left conus artery
15. Left diagonal artery (present in 33–50%)
16. Left anterior ventricular arteries
17. Anterior septal rami (supplies anterior interventricular septum)
18. Posterior septal rami
19. Left marginal artery (present in 90%)

\* Most common pattern. Shaded vessels are on posterior surface.

## Coronary Arteries

**anterior view**

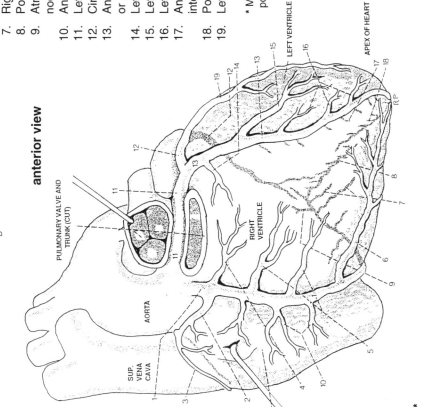

PULMONARY VALVE AND TRUNK (CUT)

AORTA

SUP. VENA CAVA

RIGHT ATRIUM

RIGHT VENTRICLE

LEFT VENTRICLE

APEX OF HEART

*after Williams and Warwick*

looking up
from below

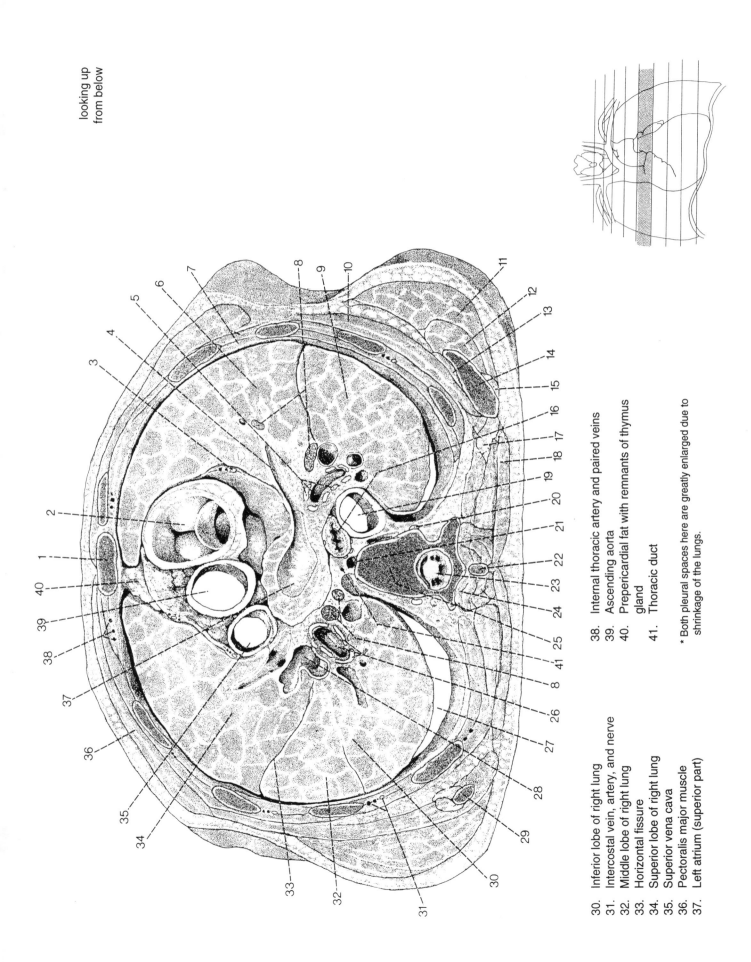

30. Inferior lobe of right lung
31. Intercostal vein, artery, and nerve
32. Middle lobe of right lung
33. Horizontal fissure
34. Superior lobe of right lung
35. Superior vena cava
36. Pectoralis major muscle
37. Left atrium (superior part)

38. Internal thoracic artery and paired veins
39. Ascending aorta
40. Prepericardial fat with remnants of thymus
    gland
41. Thoracic duct

* Both pleural spaces here are greatly enlarged due to
  shrinkage of the lungs.

# Interior of Heart

## SECTION 28
### Aortic Valve Level

*Color and label (below):*

1. Body of sternum
2. Right ventricle of heart
3. Fourth costal cartilage
4. Aortic valve (viewed from ventricular side)
5. Great cardiac vein
6. Anterior interventricular branch of left coronary artery, or left anterior descending (LAD)
7. Left ventricle (narrow outflow tract leading to aorta)
8. Wall of left ventricle
9. Superior lobe of left lung
10. Pericardium (fused with pleura)
11. Sixth intercostal vein, artery, and nerve below 6th rib (appear posterior to rib in horizontal section)
12. Portion of anterior cusp of mitral valve (bicuspid or left atrioventricular valve)
13. Lower lobe of left lung
14. Coronary sinus
15. Esophagus
16. Longissimus muscle (part of erector spinae muscle)
17. Aorta (descending thoracic part)
18. Spinal cord
19. Spinous process of vertebra T7
20. Body of thoracic vertebra T8
21. Sympathic trunk
22. Azygos vein receiving left intercostal vein
23. Right pulmonary veins emptying into left atrium
24. Left atrium
25. Latissimus dorsi muscle
26. Serratus anterior muscle
27. Pleural cavity (greatly expanded due to shrinkage of lung)
28. Middle lobe of right lung
29. Phrenic nerve, pericardiacophrenic artery and vein (between pericardium and pleura)
30. Opening of superior vena cava into right atrium

*Continued...*

*Color these veins blue or violet (below):*

1. Right brachiocephalic vein
2. Left brachiocephalic vein
3. Superior vena cava
4. Azygos vein
5. Inferior vena cava

*Color the interior of the right atrium (at left):*

6. Ostium (opening) of superior vena cava
7. Ostium of inferior vena cava
8. Ostium of coronary sinus
9. Fossa ovalis
10. Musculi pectinati
11. Crista terminalis
12. Sinoatrial node (pacemaker)
13. Right auricle

*Color the interior of the right ventricle (at left):*

14. Anterior cusp of tricuspid valve
15. Chordae tendineae
16. Anterior papillary muscle
17. Trabeculae carneae
18. Septomarginal trabecula (moderator band)
19. Conus arteriosus
20. Anterior valvule of pulmonary valve
21. Myocardium (*color pink*)
22. Endocardium (*white*)
23. Epicardium (*white*)
24. Interventricular septum
25. Pulmonary trunk
26. Right pulmonary artery
27. Left pulmonary artery
28. Superior branch of right pulmonary artery
29. Inferior branch of right pulmonary artery

*Color the left atrium (at left):*

30. Ostia (openings) of right pulmonary veins
31. Left pulmonary veins

*Color the left ventricle (at left):*

32. Anterior cusp of mitral valve
33. Posterior cusp of mitral valve
34. Chordae tendineae
35. Anterior papillary muscle
36. Left valvule of aortic valve
37. Ostium (opening) of left coronary artery
38. Aortic arch
39. Brachiocephalic artery
40. Left common carotid artery
41. Left subclavian artery

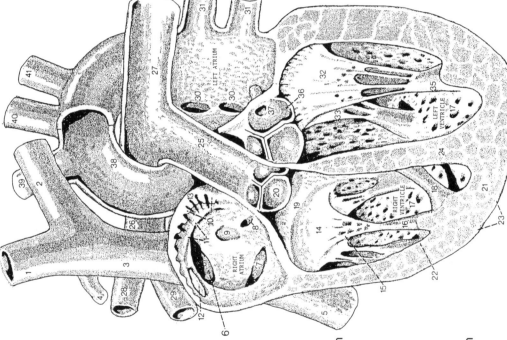

looking up
from below

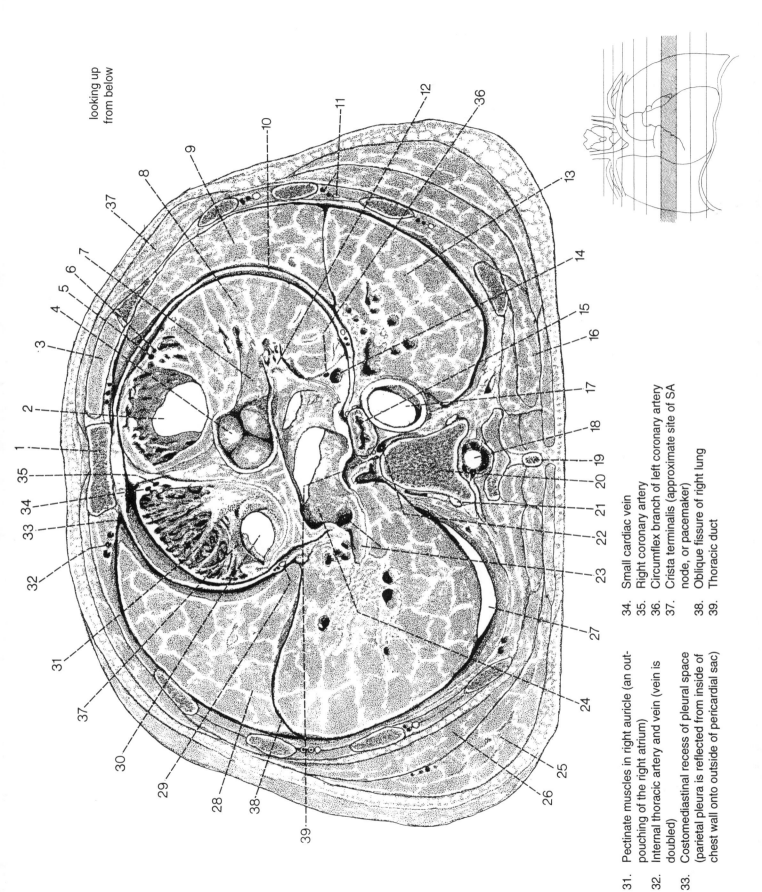

31. Pectinate muscles in right auricle (an out-
    pouching of the right atrium)
32. Internal thoracic artery and vein (vein is
    doubled)
33. Costomediastinal recess of pleural space
    (parietal pleura is reflected from inside of
    chest wall onto outside of pericardial sac)
34. Small cardiac vein
35. Right coronary artery
36. Circumflex branch of left coronary artery
37. Crista terminalis (approximate site of SA
    node, or pacemaker)
38. Oblique fissure of right lung
39. Thoracic duct

## SECTION 29
## Right and Left Ventricles Level

*Color and label:*

1. Right ventricle of heart
2. Body of sternum
3. Interventricular septum
4. Left ventricle, trabeculae carneae (muscular bundles on the inside walls of both ventricles)
5. Male nipple (papilla)
6. Anterior papillary muscle in left ventricle
7. Left phrenic nerve, pericardiacophrenic artery and vein (between pericardium and pleura)
8. Upper lobe of left lung
9. Oblique fissure in left lung
10. Chordae tendineae
11. Serratus anterior muscle
12. Anterior cusp of mitral (bicuspid) valve (left AV valve)
13. Left atrium (small portion)
14. Lower lobe of left lung
15. Coronary sinus (largest vein draining heart)
16. Descending aorta and hemiazygos vein receiving left posterior intercostal vein
17. Semispinalis (superficial) and erector spinae muscles (deep)
18. Spinal nerve T8
19. Body and lamina of thoracic vertebra T8
20. Spinal cord and internal venous plexus
21. Spinous process of thoracic vertebra T7

22. Azygos vein and right posterior intercostal vein
23. Sympathetic trunk
24. Trapezius muscle
25. Esophagus (surrounded by esophageal plexus, mainly from vagal nerve fibers) and thoracic duct
26. Latissimus dorsi muscle
27. Lower lobe of right lung
28. Intercostal vein, artery, and nerve
29. Intercostal muscles
30. Upper lobe of right lung
31. Pectoralis major muscle
32. Right atrium of heart
33. Internal thoracic artery and veins (doubled)
34. Costal cartilage
35. Anterior cusp of tricuspid valve (right AV valve)
36. Pericardium (pericardial sac—internal thin parietal serous pericardium and outer strong fibrous pericardium*
37. Posterior cusp of mitral valve
38. Enlarged pleural cavity due to lung shrinkage

* On either side the pericardium is fused with the thin parietal (or mediastinal) pleura. Phrenic nerve and accompanying vessels are "sandwiched" between pericardium and pleura.

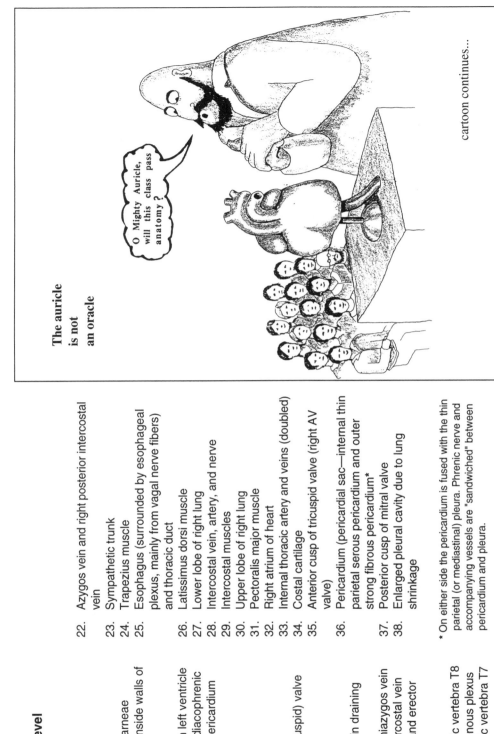

The auricle
is not
an oracle

O Mighty Auricle, will this class pass anatomy?

cartoon continues…

looking up
from below

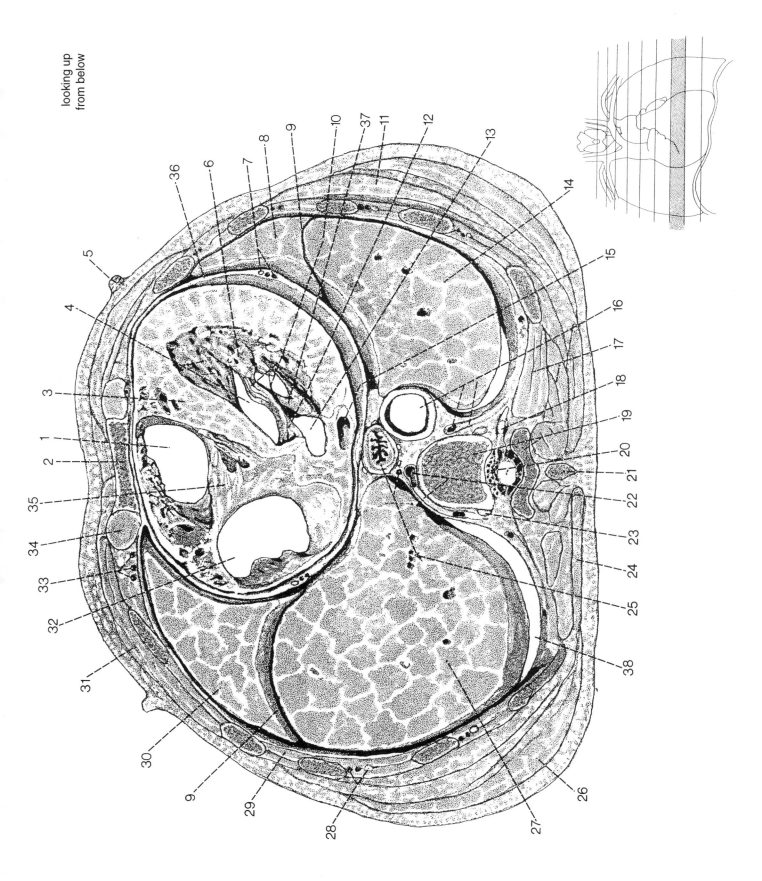

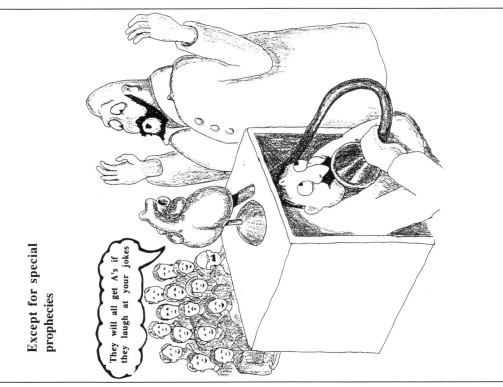

Except for special
prophecies

They will all get A's if
they laugh at your jokes

# SECTION 30
## Inferior Vena Cava, Ventricles Level

*Color and label:*

1. Inferior vena cava (arrow in right atrium points to superior lip of vena caval "half valve")
2. Thoracic aorta and thoracic duct
3. Right atrium
4. Right ventricle
5. Left ventricle
6. Esophagus (surrounded by esophageal plexus)
7. Pectoralis major muscle
8. Interventricular septum (muscular part)
9. Pleural space (actually in life a potential space containing only a little serous fluid)
10. Cusp of mitral valve
11. Lower part (lingula) of upper lobe of left lung
12. Left phrenic nerve with pericardia-cophrenic artery and vein
13. Coronary sinus (main vein draining blood from walls of heart to right atrium)
14. External and internal intercostal muscles
15. Lower lobe of left lung
16. Latissimus dorsi muscle
17. Sympathetic trunk
18. Azygos vein receiving posterior intercostal vein
19. Spinous process of thoracic vertebra T8
20. Spinal cord
21. Body of thoracic vertebra T9

22. Intercostal nerve (ventral or anterior ramus) of spinal nerve T9
23. Bare area of liver (not covered with peritoneum and firmly adhering to underside of diaphragm)
24. Right lobe of liver (its most superior part, causing right dome of diaphragm to be higher than left)
25. Diaphragm (right dome)
26. Intercostal vein (nearest to rib), artery, and nerve
27. Ninth rib
28. Serratus anterior muscle
29. Lower lobe of right lung
30. Pericardial sac (fibrous pericardium lined internally with thin serous layer and fused laterally with the pleural membrane)
31. Internal thoracic artery and vein
32. Middle lobe of right lung
33. Costal cartilage
34. Right phrenic nerve with pericardia-cophrenic artery and vein (between pericardial sac and pleura)
35. Anterior intercostal artery and vein (from internal thoracic artery)
36. Pectinate muscles in right auricle
37. Costal cartilage
38. Sternum
39. Anterior cusp and chordae tendineae of tricuspid valve

looking up
from below

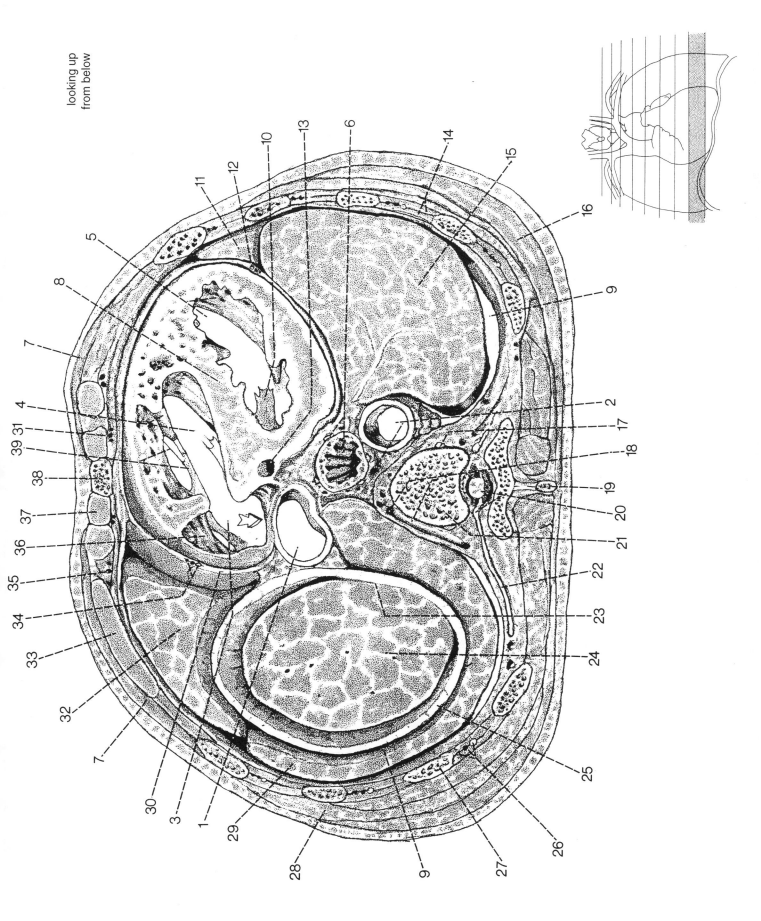

# Abdomen – Male
## Sections 31 to 40

Color and label:

1. Esophagus
2. Trachea
3. Left common carotid artery
4. Pectoralis major artery
5. Superior lobe of left lung
6. Pulmonary trunk
7. Left ventricle
8. Lower lobe of left lung
9. Stomach
10. Transverse colon
11. Rib 10
12. Descending colon
13. Ilium
14. Pubis
15. Penile (spongy) uretha
16. Spermatic cord
17. Ileocecal valve
18. Ascending colon
19. Small intestine
20. Gall bladder
21. Liver
22. Right atrium
23. Superior vena cava and opening of azygos vein
24. Aorta (ascending)
25. Brachiocephalic artery
26. Subclavian vein
27. Clavicle
28. Internal jugular vein

Frontal (Coronal) Section
of the Trunk

*after Eycleshymer and Jones*

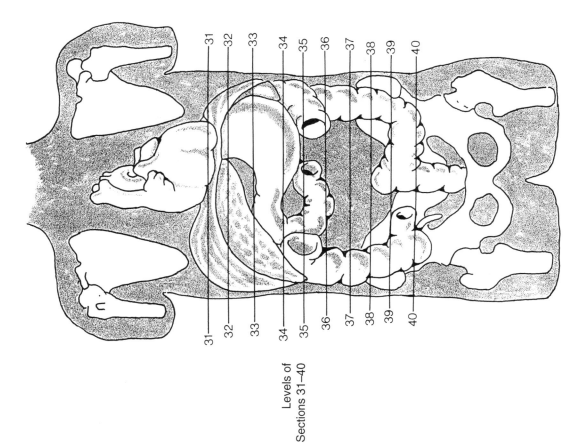

Levels of
Sections 31–40

**SECTION 31**
**Stomach Fundus Level**

*Color and label:*

1. Xiphoid process
2. Hepatogastric ligament (part of lesser omentum) within fissure for ductus venosus
3. Seventh costal cartilage
4. Sixth costal cartilage
5. Rectus abdominis muscle
6. Fifth costal cartilage
7. Inferior wall of apex of heart
8. Pericardial sac (fibrous pericardium on outside, serous parietal pericardium on inside)
9. External abdominal oblique muscle
10. Diaphragm
11. Extrapericardial fat
12. Fundus of stomach
13. Greater omentum
14. Serratus anterior muscle
15. Spleen
16. Latissimus dorsi muscle
17. Lower lobe of left lung
18. Abdominal aorta with origins of two (posterior) intercostal arteries
19. Sympathetic trunk
20. Spinal cord
21. Azygos vein
22. Thoracic duct
23. Lower lobe of right lung
24. Tenth rib
25. Inferior vena cava receiving hepatic veins
26. Caudate lobe of the liver
27. Branches of portal vein
28. Sixth rib
29. Musculophrenic artery and vein
30. Esophagus
31. Superior epigastric artery and vein
32. Right lobe of liver
33. External and internal intercostal muscles
34. Transverse process of tenth thoracic vertebra
35. Ninth rib
36. Seventh rib

looking up
from below

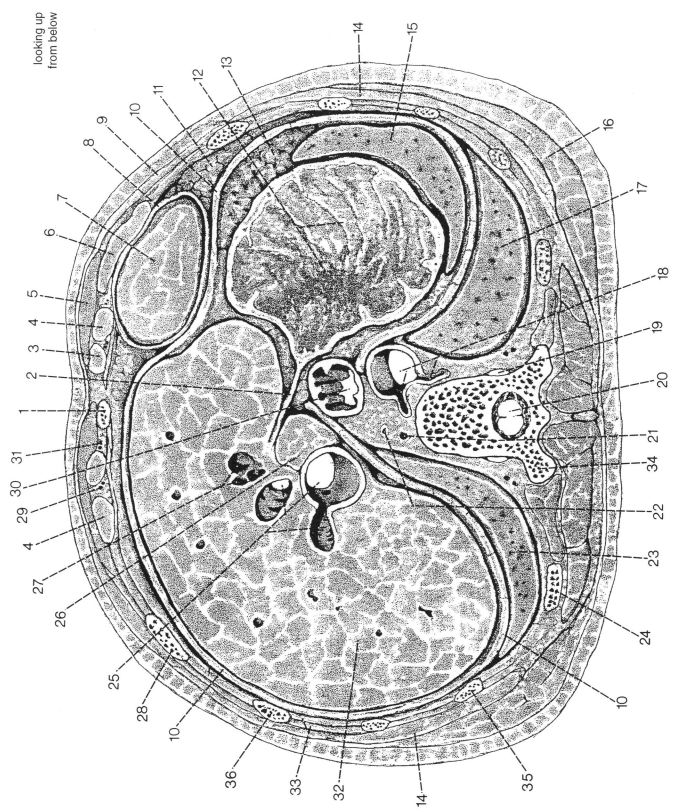

# SECTION 32
## Liver, Stomach, Spleen Level

*Color and label (below):*

1. Aorta (note beginning of a left intercostal artery)
2. Inferior vena cava
3. Esophagus
4. Stomach (fundus)
5. Stomach (body)
6. Gastric rugae (longitudinal ridges)
7. Spleen
8. Splenic vein (division)
9. Hepatic portal vein
10. Liver
11. Diaphragm
12. Transverse colon, forming splenic flexture
13. Intercostal vein, artery, and nerve
14. Descending colon, forming splenic flexture
15. Gastric vessels
16. Left and right crura of diaphragm
17. Hepatic veins
18. Ligamentum venosum (remains of ductus venosum—fetal intrahepatic continuation of umbilical vein)
19. Lesser omentum (hepatogastric ligament)
20. Costal cartilage
21. Rectus abdominis muscle
22. External abdominal oblique muscle
23. Latissimus dorsi muscle
24. Inferior surface of diaphragm (top of abdominal cavity)
25. Pleural cavity (costodiaphragmatic recess)
26. Right suprarenal gland (adrenal gland)
27. Intercostal vein and azygos vein
28. Body of thoracic vertebra T11
29. Spinal cord
30. Multifidus and spinalis muscles
31. Thoracic duct (doubled)
32. Sympathetic ganglionic chain
33. Longissimus muscle
34. Hemiazygos vein

*Color and label (at left):*

1. Greater omentum (raised up)
2. Cecum (beginning of large intestine)
3. Ascending colon
4. Transverse colon
5. Descending colon
6. Sigmoid colon
7. Jejunum (second part of small intestine)
8. Ileum (third part of small intestine)
9. Taenia coli (longitudinal strip of smooth muscle—three on large intestine)*
10. Haustra coli (outpouchings or sacculations)*
11. Appendices epiploicae (epiploic, or fatty, appendices)*

\* Found only on large intestine (colon or large bowel) and help distinguish it from small intestine.

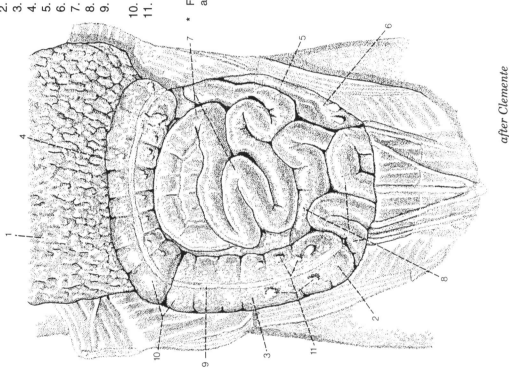

*after Clemente*

looking up
from below

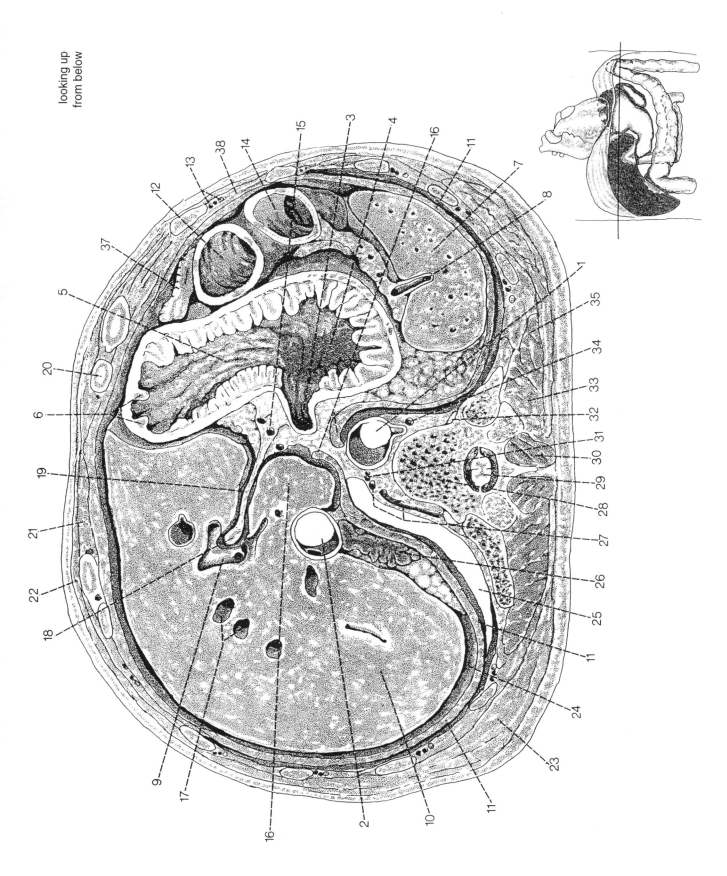

# SECTION 33
## Pancreas, Kidneys Level

*Color and label (next page):*

1. Aorta
2. Inferior vena cava
3. Portal vein
4. Common bile duct
5. Celiac trunk (see 39)
6. Common hepatic artery
7. Proper hepatic artery (origin) *
8. Splenic artery
9. Left gastric artery (origin)
10. Splenic vein
11. Spleen
12. Diaphragm
13. Stomach
14. Transverse colon (near splenic flexture)
15. Descending colon (near splenic flexture)
16. Pancreas
17. Left kidney (renal cortical substance or columns of Bertin—kidneys are normally surrounded by considerable fat)
18. Right kidney (renal pyramids— note kidneys are completely behind peritoneum or retroperitoneal)
19. Spinal cord
20. Ventral and dorsal roots of spinal nerves— course caudally and exit vertebral canal at their respective intervertebral foramina
21. Body of thoracic vertebra T12
22. Right ascending lumbar vein (usually becomes azygos vein in thorax)
23. Liver (right lobe)
24. Hepatic veins
25. External abdominal oblique muscle
26. Costal cartilage
27. Ligamentum venosum (remains of fetal ductus venosus)
28. Linea alba
29. Rectus abdominis muscle
30. Transverse mesocolon (mesentery of transverse colon)
31. Intercostal vein, artery, and nerve
32. Left ascending lumbar vein (usually becomes hemiazygos vein in thorax)

33. Longissimus muscle (part of erector spinae muscle)
34. Pleural cavity (costodiaphragmatic recess, enlarged after death)
35. Iliocostalis muscle
36. Parietal peritoneum **
37. Latissimus dorsi muscle
38. Falciform ligament
39. Origin of celiac trunk (*arrow, center*)
40. Epiploic foramen (*arrow, center left*)—opening passes ventral to inferior vena cava (2) and dorsal to the portal vein (3)
41. Suprarenal gland

\* Common hepatic artery divides at this point into the proper hepatic artery which ascends (away from viewer) and the gastroduodenal artery which descends (toward viewer).

\*\* Parietal portion of peritoneal membrane lines inner surface of abdominal walls including inferior surface of diaphragm.

*Color and label (below):*

1. Aorta
2. Celiac trunk
3. Common hepatic artery
4. Proper hepatic artery
5. Splenic artery
6. Gastroduodenal artery
7. Right gastric artery (cut)
8. Left gastric artery
9. Inferior phrenic artery
10. Common bile duct
11. Duodenum
12. Gallbladder
13. Stomach (cut)
14. Spleen
15. Pancreas
16. Superior mesenteric artery

**Celiac Trunk and Related Structures**

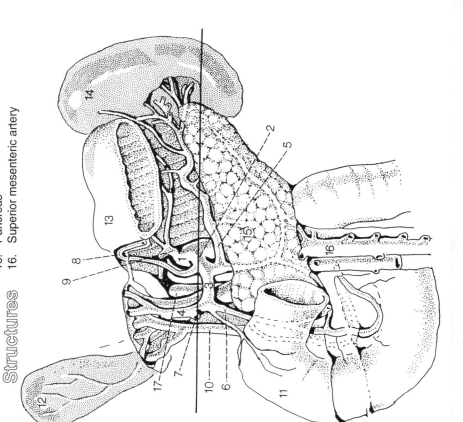
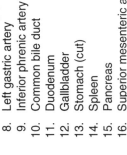
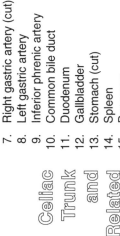
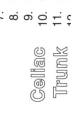
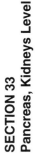

looking up
from below

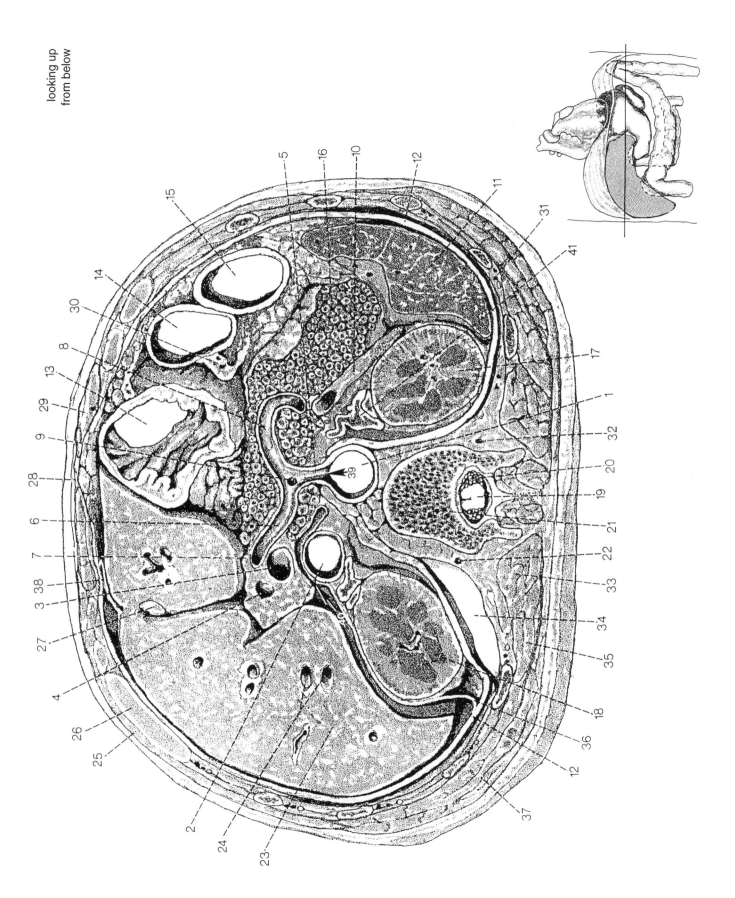

## SECTION 34
**Portal Vein Level**

*Color and label (below):*

1. Linea alba
2. Diaphragm
3. Common bile duct
4. Duodenum
5. Suprarenal gland (left)
6. Renal vein (left)
7. Intercostal vein, artery, and nerve
8. Rectus abdominis muscle
9. Stomach
10. Portal vein
11. Superior mesenteric artery
12. Transverse colon
13. Pancreas (body and tail)
14. Descending colon
15. Spleen
16. Renal artery
17. Left kidney
18. Left crus of diaphragm
19. Iliocostalis muscle
20. Psoas major muscle
21. Aorta
22. Body of lumbar vertebra L1
23. Conus medullaris of spinal cord and cauda equina
24. Multifidus muscle
25. Longissimus muscle
26. Quadratus lumborum muscle
27. Right crus of diaphragm
28. Inferior vena cava and right and left renal veins
29. Right kidney (renal pyramid)
30. Latissimus dorsi muscle
31. Liver (right lobe)
32. Gall bladder
33. Costal cartilage
34. External abdominal oblique muscle
35. Liver (left lobe)
36. Round ligament (ligamentum teres) of the liver (remains of umbilical vein)
37. Falciform ligament
38. Pancreas (head)

## Stomach, Duodenum, and Pancreas

*Color and label (at left):*

1. Esophagus
2. Cardiac orifice and cardiac region of stomach
3. Fundus of stomach
4. Body of stomach
5. Pyloric antrum
6. Pyloric canal
7. Pyloric opening
8. Pyloric sphincter muscle (*pylorus*—Gr., gatekeeper)
9. Duodenum (first, superior part—duodenal bulb)
10. Duodenum (second, descending part)
11. Duodenum (third, horizontal part)
12. Duodenum (fourth, ascending part)
13. Probe in greater duodenal papilla (opening of common bile duct and pancreatic duct)
14. Lesser duodenal papilla (opening of accessory pancreatic duct)
15. Pancreatic duct (head of pancreas partially removed)
16. Accessory pancreatic duct
17. Head of pancreas (cut)
18. Circular folds in duodenum (plicae ciruclares)
19. Common bile duct
20. Cystic duct
21. Common hepatic duct
22. Right hepatic duct
23. Left hepatic duct
24. Gallbladder
25. Gastric ridges (*gaster*—Gr., stomach or belly)
26. Aorta (abdominal)
27. Celiac trunk
28. Left gastric artery
29. Splenic artery
30. Common heptaic artery
31. Proper hepatic artery
32. Left hepatic artery
33. Right hepatic artery
34. Middle hepatic artery
35. Right gastric artery
36. Gastroduodenal artery
37. Superior mesenteric vein
38. Superior mesenteric artery

looking up
from below

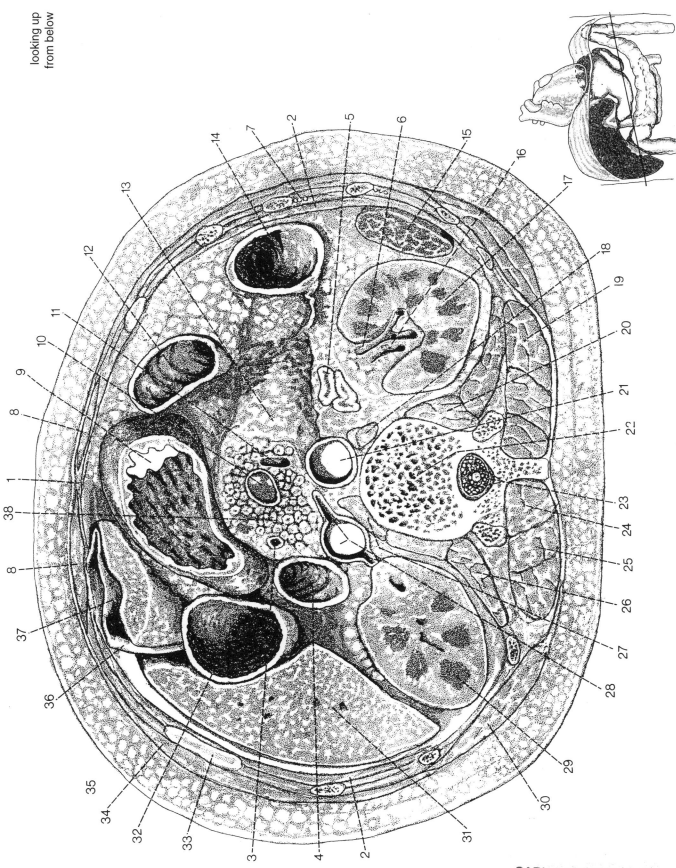

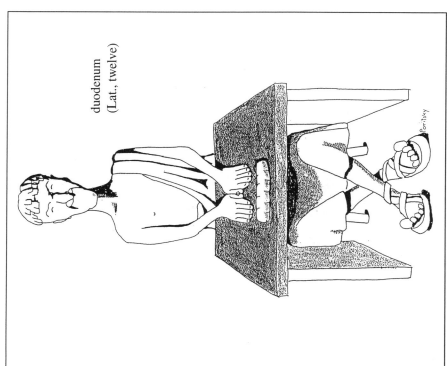

duodenum
(Lat., twelve)

**The Latin twelve refers to twelve fingerbreadths.** The duodenum was so named because it is supposedly as long as twelve fingers placed side by side. Thus the duodenum, which is the first part of the small intestine, is only about ten inches long.

## SECTION 35
## Transverse Colon Level

*Color and label:*

1. Aorta with lumbar arteries
2. Inferior vena cava with right testicular vein
3. Superior mesenteric vein
4. Superior mesenteric artery
5. Jejunum
6. Transverse colon
7. Right colic (hepatic) flexure (bend at end of ascending colon and beginning of transverse colon)
8. Descending colon
9. Duodenum (second, descending part)
10. Bristle in major duodenal papilla
11. Duodenum (fourth, ascending part), transition to jejunum
12. Liver (right lobe)
13. Gall bladder (bottom surface)
14. Right kidney
15. Left kidney
16. Cauda equina (roots of lower lumbar nerves L3–L5, sacral nerves S1–S5, and coccygeal nerve)
17. Nucleus pulposus of intervertebral disk between lumbar vertebrae L2 and L3
18. Annulus (anulus) fibrosus of intervertebral disk L2–L3
19. Left testicular vein
20. Psoas major muscle
21. Spinous process of vertebra L2
22. Inferior mesenteric vein
23. Perirenal fat
24. Left ureter
25. Rectus abdominis muscle
26. Greater omentum
27. Linea alba
28. Falciform ligament
29. Inferior epigastric artery and vein (these vessels often divide into two or more collateral branches)
30. Round ligament of liver (remains of umbilical vein)
31. External abdominal oblique muscle
32. Internal abdominal oblique muscle
33. Transversus abdominis muscle
34. Eleventh rib
35. Twelfth rib
36. Latissimus dorsi muscle
37. Right ureter
38. Iliocostalis muscle
39. Quadratus lumborum muscle
40. Longissimus muscle
41. Dorsal root ganglion of lumbar nerve L2
42. Multifidus and spinalis muscles

looking up
from below

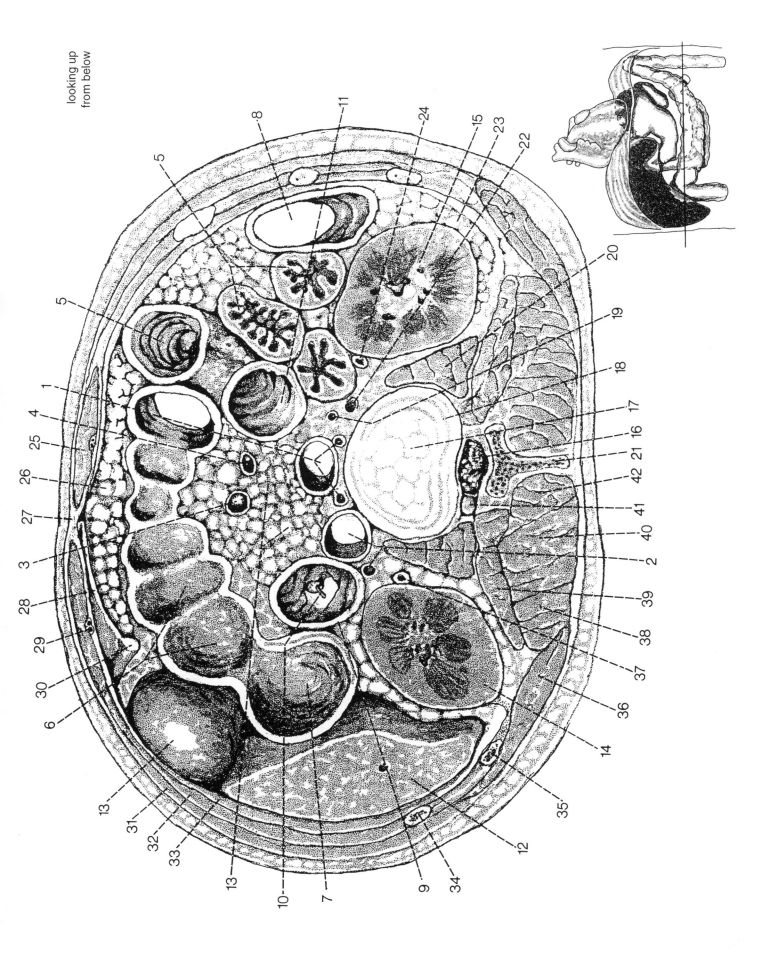

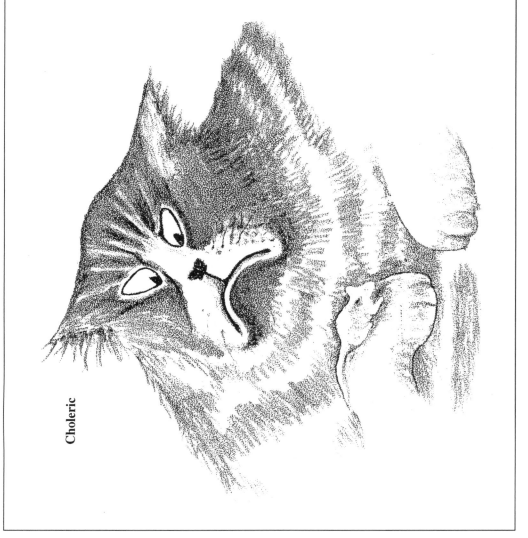

**Choleric**

**Greek for "yellow bile" was *chole*,** and supposedly too much yellow bile would render one choleric, or hot-tempered, angry, irate, irascible. The ancient Greeks believed that there were four body fluids, or as they were later called, four humors, which, in varying proportions, determined temperament. An abundance on one humor would bestow upon an individual a certain disposition (we say "personality").

Fresh bile or gall is a golden yellow; on exposure to air it turns greenish black. This misled the ancient Greeks into believing that there were two kinds of bile, yellow and black.

**SECTION 36**
**Duodenum (3rd Part) Level**

*Color and label:*

1. Superior mesenteric vein
2. Linea alba
3. Superior mesenteric artery
4. Inferior epigastric artery and vein
5. Greater omentum
6. Circular folds (Lat., plicae circulares), formerly valves of Kerckring
7. Jejunum
8. Transversus abdominis muscle
9. Internal abdominal oblique muscle
10. External abdominal oblique muscle
11. Left testicular artery and vein
12. Inferior mesenteric vein
13. Descending colon
14. Left ureter
15. Left kidney (inferior pole)
16. Quadratus lumborum muscle
17. Psoas major muscle
18. Iliocostalis muscle
19. Aorta
20. Body of lumbar vertebra L3
21. Multifidus muscle
22. Cauda equina
23. Dorsal root ganglion of lumbar nerve L3
24. Inferior vena cava
25. Right ureter
26. Latissimus dorsi muscle
27. Right kidney (inferior pole)
28. Right testicular vein
29. Right lobe of liver (inferior part)
30. Ascending colon
31. Transverse colon
32. Third (horizontal) part of duodenum
33. Rectus abdominis muscle

looking up from below

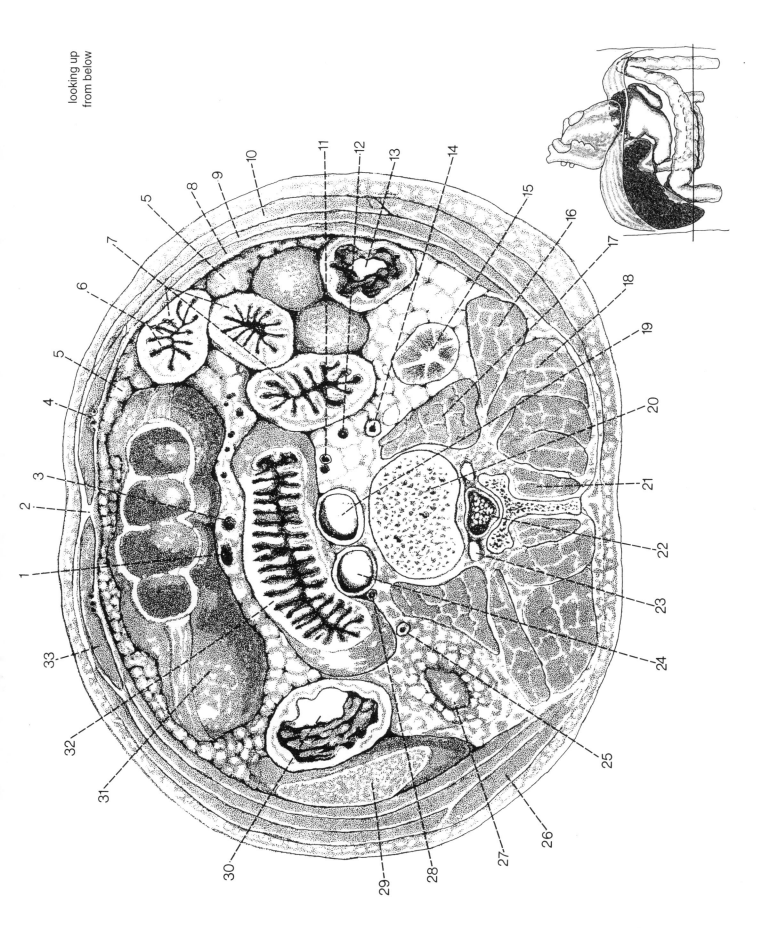

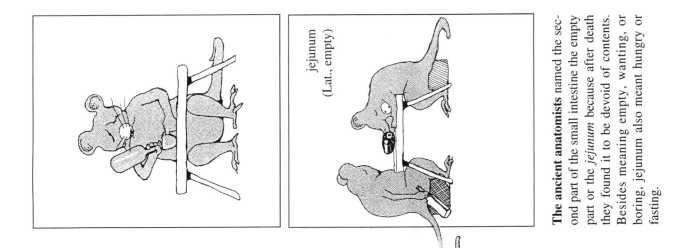

jejunum
(Lat., empty)

**The ancient anatomists** named the second part of the small intestine the empty part or the *jejunum* because after death they found it to be devoid of contents. Besides meaning empty, wanting, or boring, jejunum also meant hungry or fasting.

## SECTION 37
## Iliac Crest, Jejunum Level

*Color and label:*

1. Inferior vena cava
2. Rectus abdominis muscle
3. Branches of superior mesenteric artery and vein in mesentery
4. Linea alba
5. Aorta
6. Inferior mesenteric artery (next to aorta) and vein
7. Superior epigastric artery and vein
8. Greater omentum
9. Exteral abdominal oblique muscle
10. Internal abdominal oblique muscle
11. Transversus abdominis muscle
12. Descending colon
13. Jejunum
14. Iliac crest
15. Psoas major muscle
16. Third lumbar nerve (L3)
17. Vertebral venous plexus
18. Cauda equina within dural sheath
19. Anterior longitudinal ligament
20. Lumbar sympathetic chain
21. Right ureter
22. Right testicular artery and vein
23. Quadratus lumborum muscle
24. Ascending colon
25. Lumbar vertebra L4 (body)

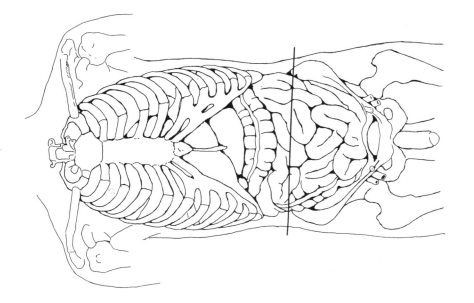

looking up
from below

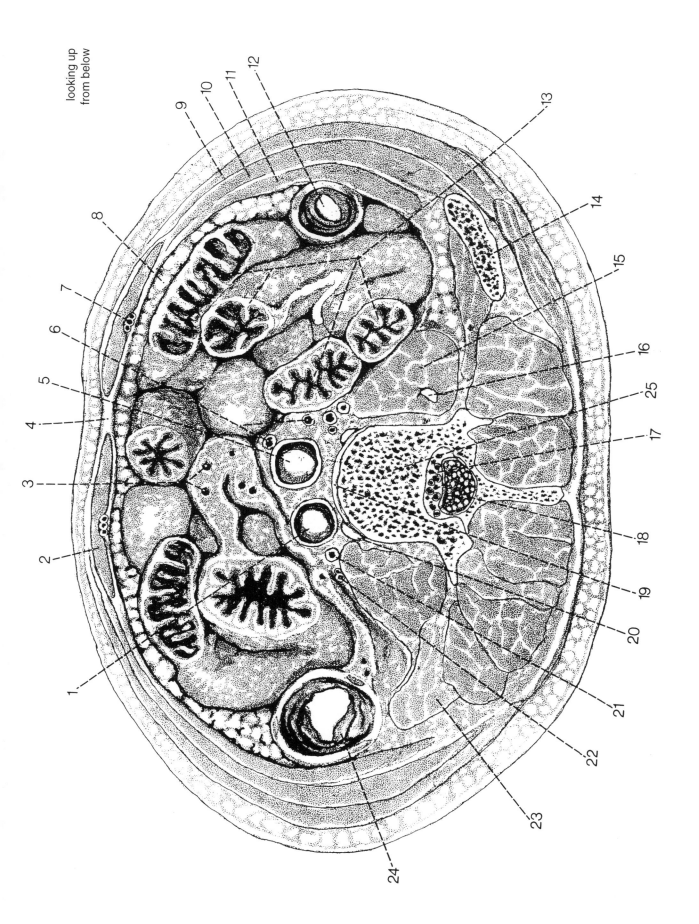

**Melancholic**

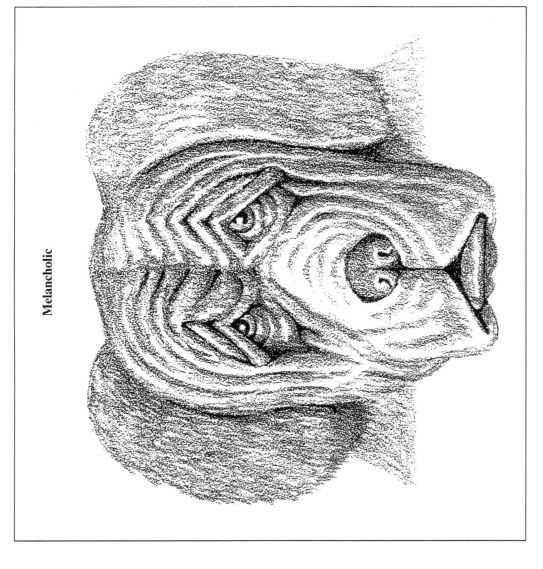

**SECTION 38**
**Umbilicus Level**

*Color and label:*

1. Inferior vena cava
2. Anterior layer of rectus sheath
3. Aorta
4. Linea alba
5. Umbilicus
6. Superior rectal artery
7. Superior rectal vein
8. Inferior epigastric artery and vein(s)
9. Lymph nodes in mesentery
10. Rectus abdominis muscle
11. Jejunum (second part of small intestine)
12. External abdominal oblique muscle
13. Internal abdominal oblique muscle
14. Transversus abdominis muscle
15. Descending colon
16. Deep circumflex iliac artery and vein
17. Left testicular artery and vein
18. Psoas major muscle
19. Ureter (left)
20. Intervertebral disk between L4 and L5
21. Dural sac containing cauda equina
22. Body of vertebra L4
23. Lumbar nerve L3 in psoas major muscle
24. Ureter (right)
25. Right testicular artery and vein
26. Ilium (part of hip bone or coxal bone)
27. Gluteus medius muscle
28. Iliacus muscle
29. Ascending colon
30. Ileum (third part of small intestine)

**Greek for "black bile" was *melancholy*,** one of the four humors. An oversupply of black bile would make one sad or melancholy. Clinical melancholia is a mental disorder with symptoms very much like those described two thousand years ago. Melanin is the black pigment in the skin. *Melanesia* is Greek for "black island" (*melas, melanos*—"black" + *nesos*—"island").

looking up
from below

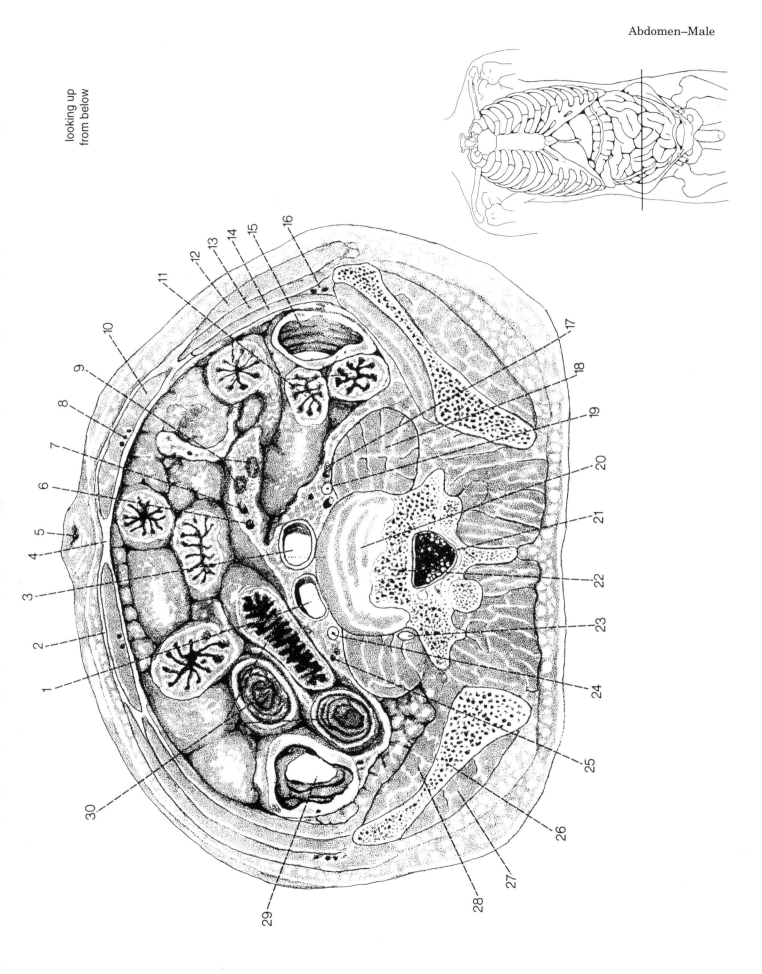

**Phlegmatic**

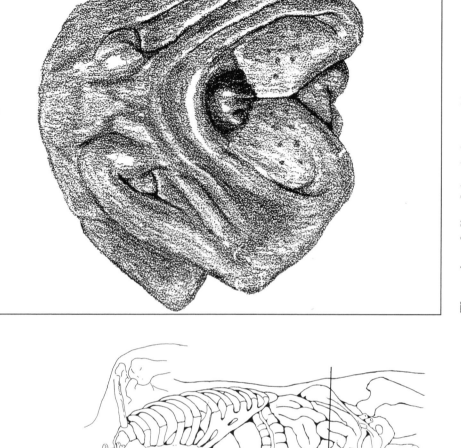

**The ancients believed** that the humor phlegm was extracted from the blood by the brain, conveyed to the pituitary gland, and hence to the nose. Too much phlegm would make one phlegmatic. "Phlegm" is now the name for the viscous mucus coughed up from the lungs. A phlegmatic personality refers to a person who is slow or sluggish. In this respect, the term retains its original meaning.

## SECTION 39
## Common Iliac Vessels Level

*Color and label:*

1. Ascending colon
2. Ileum
3. Right and left common iliac veins
4. Rectus abdominis muscle
5. Inferior epigastric artery and vein(s)
6. Right and left common iliac arteries
7. Linea alba
8. Inferior mesenteric vessels
9. Anterior layer of rectus sheath
10. Greater omentum
11. Jejunum
12. Testicular artery and vein
13. Descending colon
14. Transversus abdominis muscle
15. Internal abdominal oblique muscle
16. External abdominal oblique muscle
17. Deep circumflex iliac artery and vein
18. Gluteus minimus muscle
19. Iliacus muscle
20. Ilium (part of coxal or hip bone)
21. Ureter
22. Gluteus medius muscle
23. Gluteus maximus muscle
24. Inferior gluteal artery, vein, and nerve
25. Body of first sacral segment
26. Roots of sacral nerves (descending within dural sheath) and part of cauda equina
27. Multifidus muscle
28. Posterior superior iliac spine
29. Lateral mass (ala) of first sacral segment
30. Psoas major muscle
31. Superior gluteal artery, vein, and nerve
32. Anterior superior iliac spine
33. Femoral nerve
34. Sacro-iliac joint

looking up
from below

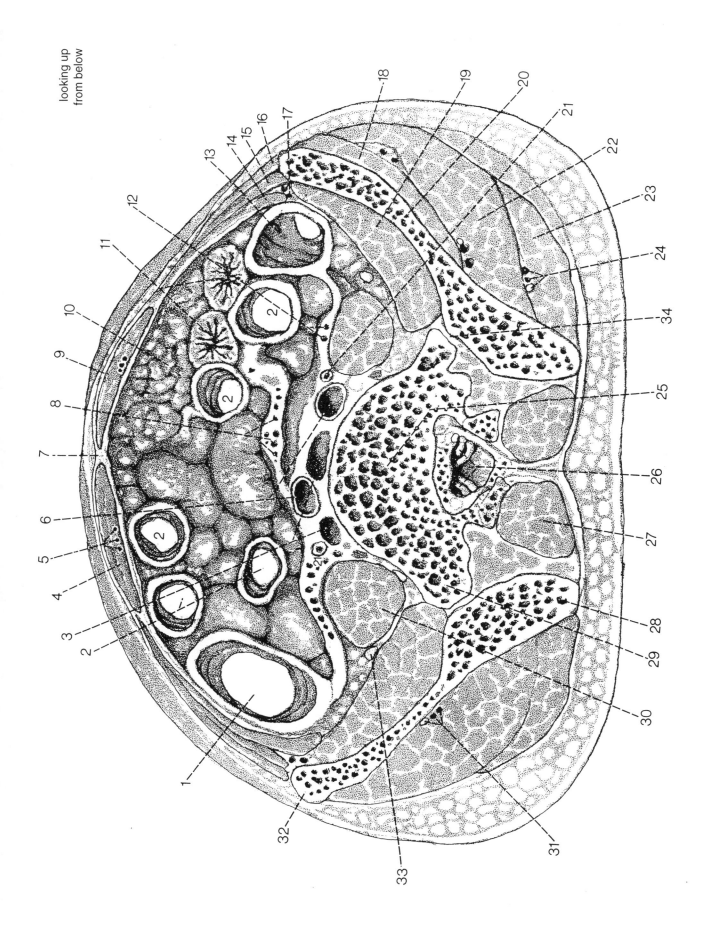

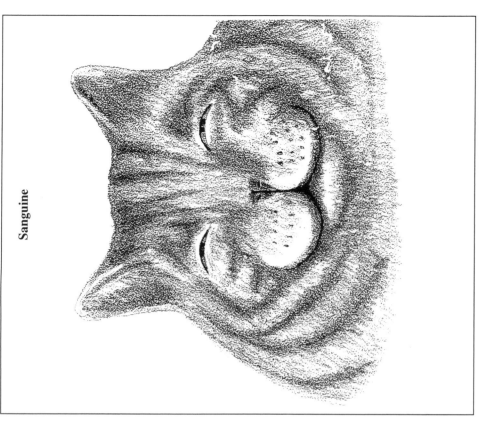

Sanguine

**Sanguine means "cheerful" and "optimistic."** The ancients believed this was due to an abundance of *sanguis* or blood. The Greek term for blood is *haima*, which has given us "hematology" (study of blood) and related terms. The definition of sanguine is similar today, except it no longer includes "a ruddy complexion." Sanguinary, on the other hand, means bloodthirsty and murderous; so one shouldn't confuse the two terms.

**SECTION 40**
**Ileum Level**

*Color and label:*

1. Ascending colon
2. Ureter (right and left)
3. Ileum
4. Inferior epigastric artery and vein
5. Mesentery of ileum
6. Linea alba
7. Jejunum (partially cut—note abundant circular folds)
8. Rectus abdominis muscle
9. Greater omentum
10. Testicular artery and vein
11. Descending colon
12. Genitofemoral nerve
13. Left external iliac artery
14. Femoral nerve
15. Gluteus minimus muscle
16. Iliacus muscle
17. Left external iliac vein
18. Ilium
19. Left internal iliac artery
20. Obturator nerve
21. Left internal iliac vein
22. Lumbosacral trunk
23. Sacrum
24. Sacral canal
25. Multifidus muscle
26. Right internal iliac artery
27. Sacro-iliac joint
28. Right common iliac vein (origin)
29. Right external iliac artery
30. Gluteus medius muscle
31. Gluteus maximus muscle
32. Deep circumflex iliac vessels and ilioinguinal nerve
33. Inferior gluteal artery and vein
34. Psoas major muscle

looking up
from below

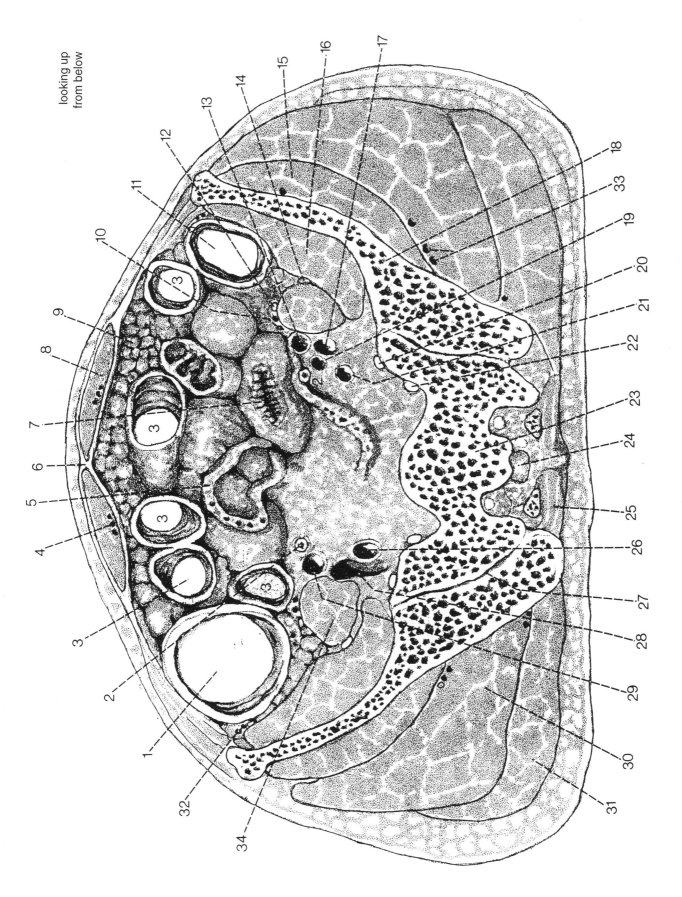

*Testis* **means "witness" in Latin,** and *testicle* means "little witness." There seem to be several theories to account for the word's origin. The testes testify to one's manhood, and only men could give witness or testify in an ancient Roman court of law or forum. Professor William Haubrich* writes that in certain ancient cultures, when giving testimony the witness or testifier grasped the scrotum, presumably his own, but on occasion someone else's. In Genesis 24:9 there is a passage in which Abraham's servant places his hand on his master's scrotum while swearing an oath.

The Romans used the term in the sense of "lookers-on" or "peepers," since the testes are in a position to observe the sexual act close up.

\* William Haubrich, *Medical Meanings.* Harcourt, Brace, and Jovanovich, San Diego, 1984.

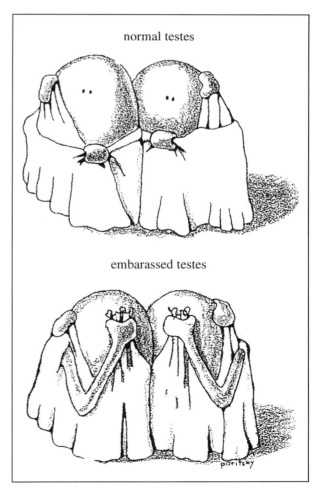

normal testes

embarassed testes

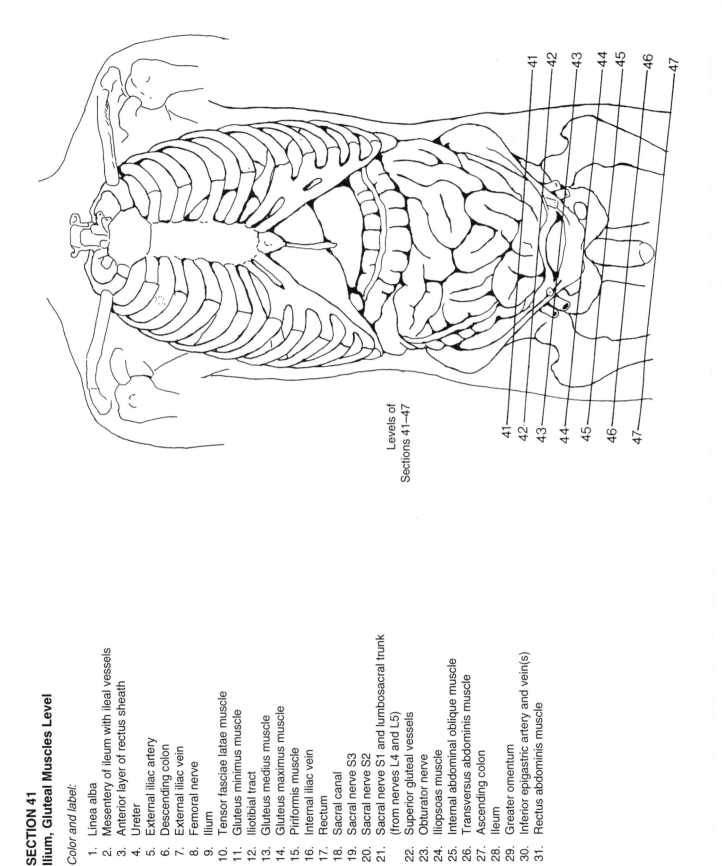

**SECTION 41**
**Ilium, Gluteal Muscles Level**

*Color and label:*

1. Linea alba
2. Mesentery of ileum with ileal vessels
3. Anterior layer of rectus sheath
4. Ureter
5. External iliac artery
6. Descending colon
7. External iliac vein
8. Femoral nerve
9. Ilium
10. Tensor fasciae latae muscle
11. Gluteus minimus muscle
12. Iliotibial tract
13. Gluteus medius muscle
14. Gluteus maximus muscle
15. Piriformis muscle
16. Internal iliac vein
17. Rectum
18. Sacral canal
19. Sacral nerve S3
20. Sacral nerve S2
21. Sacral nerve S1 and lumbosacral trunk
    (from nerves L4 and L5)
22. Superior gluteal vessels
23. Obturator nerve
24. Iliopsoas muscle
25. Internal abdominal oblique muscle
26. Transversus abdominis muscle
27. Ascending colon
28. Ileum
29. Greater omentum
30. Inferior epigastric artery and vein(s)
31. Rectus abdominis muscle

Levels of
Sections 41–47

looking up
from below

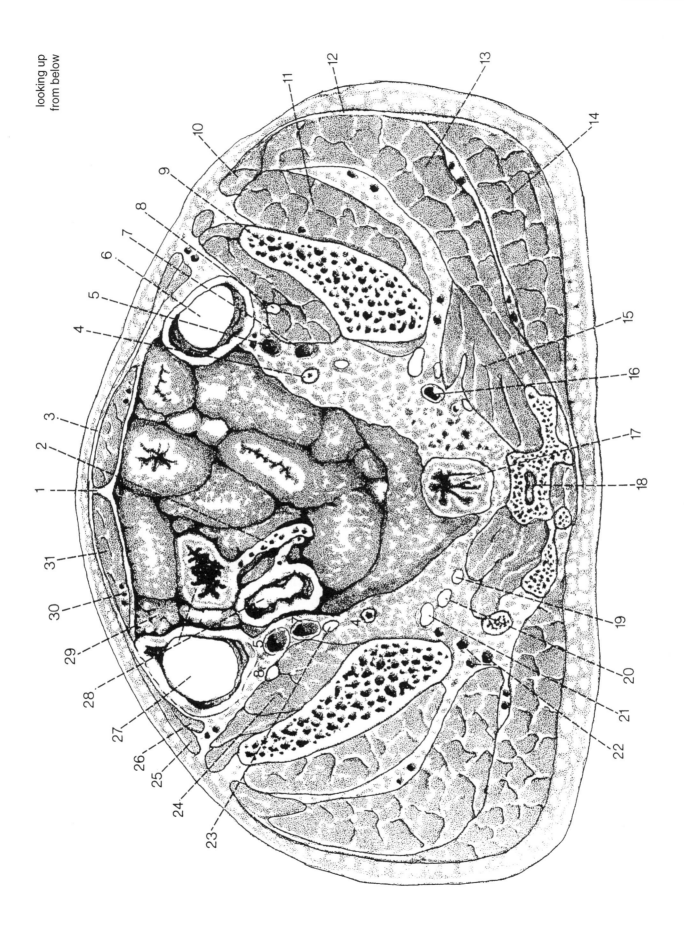

## Male Pelvis

*Color and label (at left):*

1. Skin
2. Superficial (fatty) layer of superficial fascia (Camper's)
3. Deep membranous layer of superficial fascia (Scarpa's)
4. Dartos tunic—sheet of smooth muscle comprising superficial fascia of scrotum
5. Skin of scrotum
6. Testis (covered with tunica vaginalis)
7. Epididymis
8. Parietal layer (cut) of tunica vaginalis testis
9. Testicular vein forming pampiniform plexus
10. Ductus (vas) deferens
11. Superior ramus of pubic bone
12. Ramus of ischium
13. Membranous layer of superficial fascia
14. Puborectalis muscle (part of levator ani muscle)
15. Levator ani muscle
16. Rectum
17. Peritoneum (cut edge)
18. Prostate gland
19. Bladder
20. Seminal vesicle
21. Ureter (cut)
22. Superficial fascia of penis
23. Corpus cavernosus penis
24. Corpus spongiosum
25. Prepuce of penis
26. Glans
27. External anal sphincter

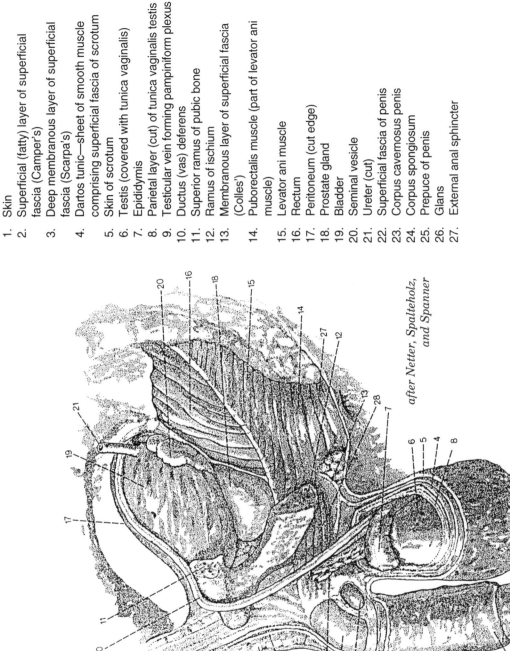

*after Netter, Spalteholz, and Spanner*

## SECTION 42
## Cecum, Head of Femur, and Acetabulum Level

*Color and label (below):*

1. Linea alba
2. Jejunum
3. Inferior epigastric artery and vein(s)
4. Sigmoid colon
5. Testicular vessels
6. Lymph node
7. Deep circumflex iliac vessels
8. Femoral nerve
9. Iliofemoral ligament
10. Head of femur
11. Obturator internus muscle
12. Piriformis muscle
13. Inferior gluteal vessels
14. Pudendal nerve, internal pudendal vessels

*Continued...*

looking up
from below

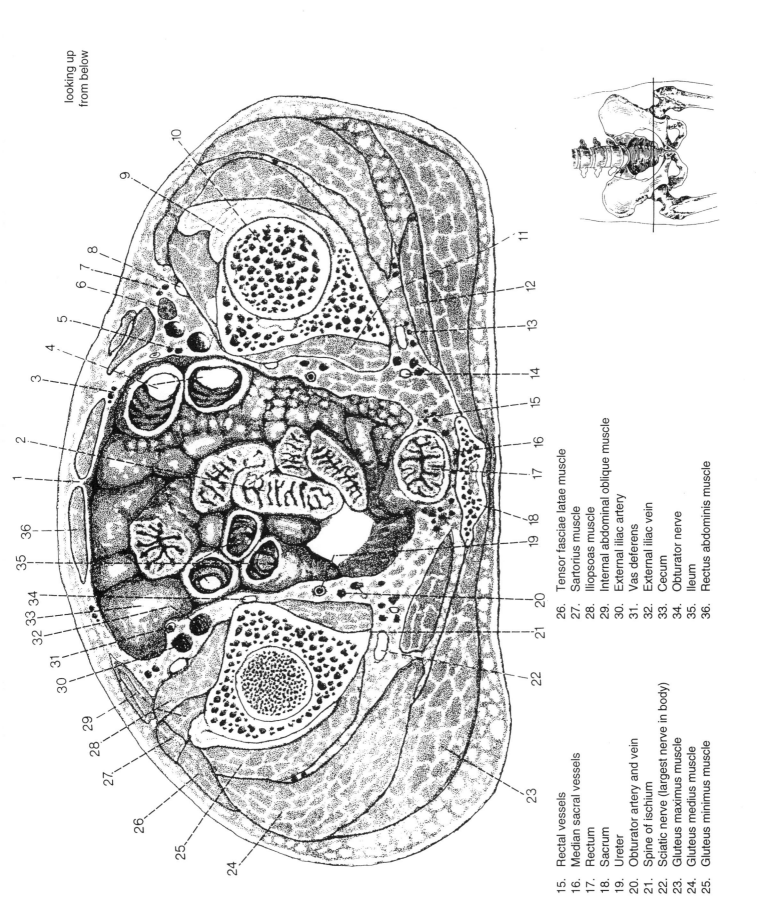

15. Rectal vessels
16. Median sacral vessels
17. Rectum
18. Sacrum
19. Ureter
20. Obturator artery and vein
21. Spine of ischium
22. Sciatic nerve (largest nerve in body)
23. Gluteus maximus muscle
24. Gluteus medius muscle
25. Gluteus minimus muscle

26. Tensor fasciae latae muscle
27. Sartorius muscle
28. Iliopsoas muscle
29. Internal abdominal oblique muscle
30. External iliac artery
31. Vas deferens
32. External iliac vein
33. Cecum
34. Obturator nerve
35. Ileum
36. Rectus abdominis muscle

# SECTION 43
## Spermatic Cord, Seminal Vesicles Level

*Color and label (next page):*

1. Linea alba
2. Rectus abdominis muscle within tendinous sheath
3. Urinary bladder (internal surface of superior half)
4. Left spermatic cord
5. Pectineus muscle
6. Pubis
7. Ligament of femoral head (formerly round ligament of femur)
8. Sartorius muscle
9. Head of femur
10. Iliofemoral ligament
11. Tensor fascia lata muscle
12. Gluteus medius muscle
13. Iliotibial tract
14. Greater trochanter
15. Neck of femur
16. Inferior gemellus muscle
17. Tendon of obturator internus muscle
18. Inferior gluteal artery and vein
19. Superior gemellus muscle
20. Spine of ischium
21. Sacrospinous ligament and coccygeus muscle
22. Rectum
23. Coccyx
24. Ductus (vas) deferens
25. Seminal vesicle
26. Pudendal nerve, internal pudendal artery and vein
27. Gluteus maximus muscle
28. Sciatic nerve
29. Head of femur within acetabulum
30. Superior tip of right greater trochanter
31. Ischiofemoral ligament
32. Gluteus medius muscle
33. Gluteus minimus muscle
34. Rectus femoris muscle (part of quadriceps femoris muscle)

*Continued...*

*Color and label (below):*

1. Pubic symphysis
2. Bladder
3. Rectum
4. Ejactulatory duct
5. Prostate gland
6. Bulbourethral gland (of Cowper)
7. Bulbospongiosus muscle
8. Septum of scrotum
9. Prepuce (foreskin)
10. Glans of penis
11. Urethra
12. Corpus spongiosus of penis
13. Corpus cavernosum of penis

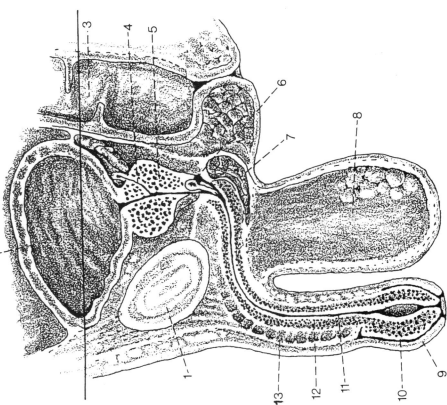

Male Pelvis, Median Section

looking up
from below

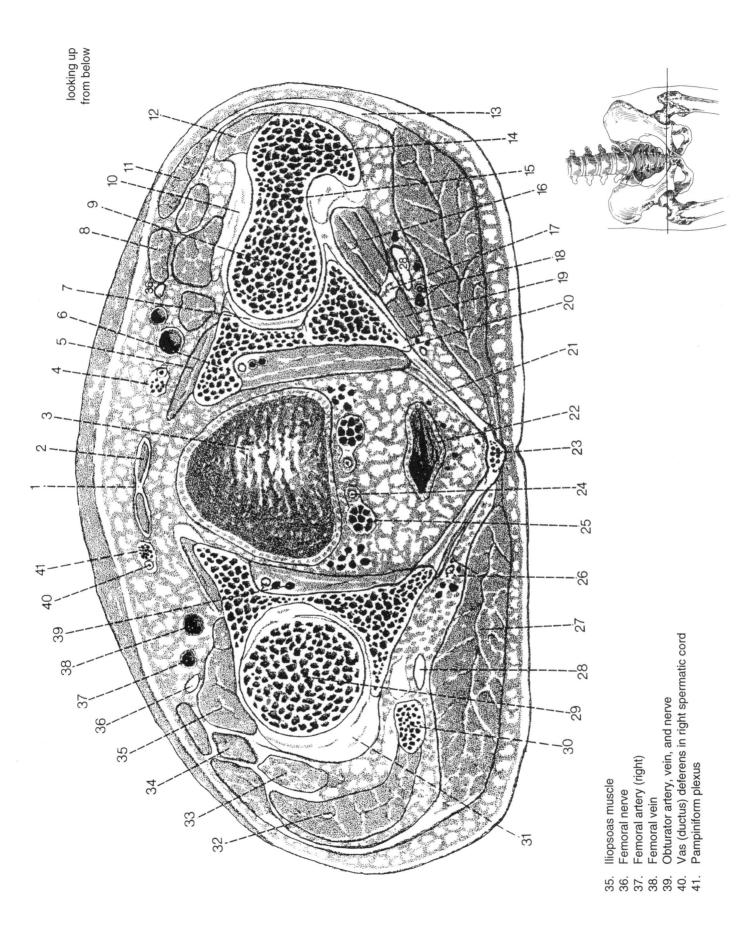

35. Iliopsoas muscle
36. Femoral nerve
37. Femoral artery (right)
38. Femoral vein
39. Obturator artery, vein, and nerve
40. Vas (ductus) deferens in right spermatic cord
41. Pampiniform plexus

## SECTION 44
### Prostate Gland, Obturator Foramen Level

*Color and label (below):*

1. Pubic symphysis
2. Pubis (part of superior ramus)
3. Vas deferens in left spermatic cord
4. Adductor longus muscle
5. Obturator membrane
6. Obturator externus muscle
7. Deep (profunda) femoral artery
8. Lateral femoral circumflex artery
9. Medial femoral circumflex artery and vein
10. Iliopsoas muscle and tendon
11. Vastus lateralis muscle
12. Iliotibial tract
13. Left femur
14. Quadratus femoris muscle
15. Sciatic nerve and inferior gluteal vessels
16. Obturator internus muscle
17. Pudendal nerve, internal pudendal artery and vein
18. Prostate gland
19. Puborectalis muscle
20. Rectum
21. Prostatic urethra
22. Right ischial tuberosity
23. Gluteus maximus muscle
24. Medial circumflex femoral vessels
25. Right femur
26. Tensor fascia lata muscle
27. Lateral circumflex femoral artery and vein (ascending branches)
28. Rectus femoris muscle
29. Lesser trochanter
30. Sartorius muscle
31. Right femoral nerve
32. Deep femoral artery
33. Right femoral artery
34. Right femoral vein
35. Great saphenous vein
36. Pectineus muscle

*Continued...*

## Scrotum and Spermatic Cord

*Color and label (at left):*

1. Spermatic cord
2. Ductus deferens
3. Epididymis (head)
4. Pampiniform plexus (drains into testicular vein)*
5. Testicular artery
6. Ductus deferens artery (arises from patent part of umbilical artery)
7. Testis (covered with visceral layer of tunica vaginalis)
8. Superficial inguinal ring
9. Ilioguinal nerve
10. Genitofemoral nerve (genital branch—supplies cremaster muscle)
11. Tunica vaginalis (parietal layer)
12. External spermatic fascia
13. Cremasteric fascia and muscle
14. Internal spermatic fascia
15. Epididymis (isolated with efferent ductules)
16. Testis (sectioned with lobules)
17. Skin of scrotum
18. Dartos tunic (smooth muscle)
19. Septum of scrotum

* Acts as counter–current heat exhanger with testicular artery, thus cooling arterial blood heading to testes

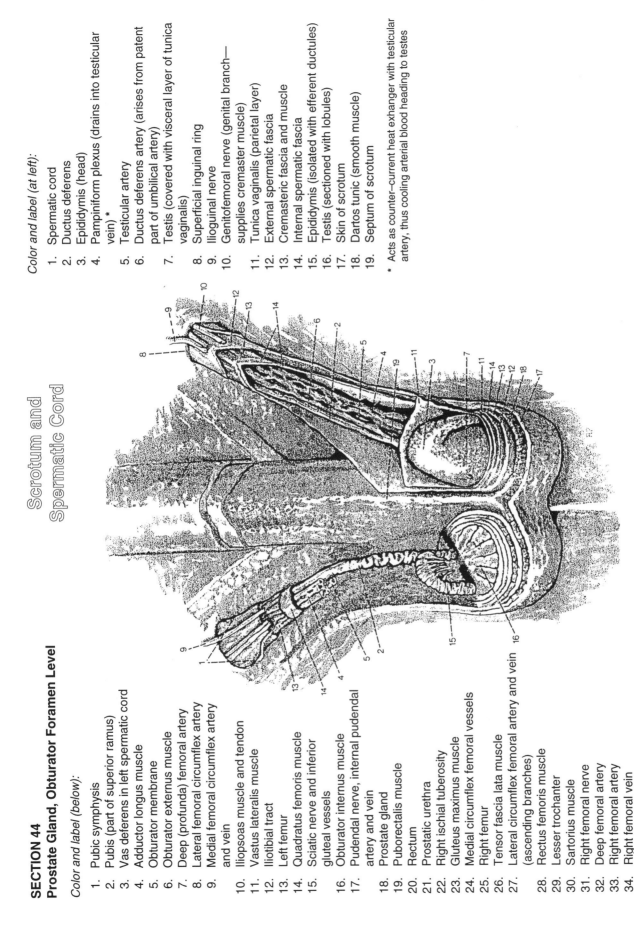

looking up
from below

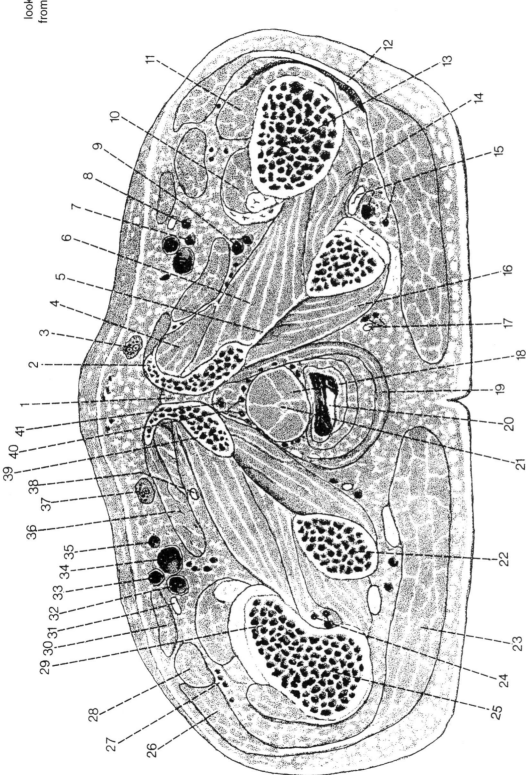

37. Right spermatic cord
38. Obturator nerve
39. Pubis (inferior ramus)
40. Prostatic venous plexus
41. Dorsal vein of penis

# SECTION 45
## Penis, Spermatic Cord Level

*Color and label (below):*

1. Pampiniform (venous) plexus
2. Dorsal vessels of penis
3. Corpus cavernosus of penis
4. Spermatic cord
5. Vas (ductus) deferens
6. Gracilis muscle (mainly tendinous in this section)
7. Adductor longus muscle
8. Inguinal lymph node
9. Great saphenous vein
10. Femoral vein
11. Femoral artery
12. Femoral nerve
13. Deep (profunda) femoral artery
14. Lateral circumflex femoral artery and vein
15. Tensor fascia lata muscle
16. Iliopsoas muscle and tendon
17. Vastus intermedius muscle
18. Vastus lateralis muscle
19. Femur (shaft)
20. Quadratus femoris muscle
21. Gluteus maximus muscle
22. Obturator externus muscle
23. Ischiorectal fossa (filled with fat)
24. Urethra (spongy)
25. Levator ani muscle
26. Anal canal
27. Bulb of penis
28. Ischium
29. Semitendinosus muscle (tendon)
30. Biceps femoris muscle (long head, tendon)
31. Semimembranosus muscle (tendon)
32. Inferior gluteal artery, vein, and nerve
33. Sciatic nerve *
34. Lesser trochanter of femur
35. Iliotibial tract
36. Medial circumflex femoral artery and vein

\* Actually a double nerve: the lateral half is the common peroneal; the medial half is the tibial nerve.

*Continued....*

*Color and label (at left):*

1. Testis
2. Epididymis (Gr., upon the twin, i.e., the testes)
3. Ductus deferens
4. Bladder
5. Seminal vesicle
6. Ureter (cut)
7. Ejaculatory duct (common duct for ductus deferens and seminal vesicle—conveys semen to urethra)
8. Prostate gland
9. Prostatic urethra
10. Urethral sphincter muscle
11. Bulbourethral glands
12. Bulb of penis and bulbospongiosus muscle
13. Left crus of penis and ischiocavernosus muscle
14. Right crus of penis (cut showing cavernous spaces in erectile tissue)
15. Site of attachment to ischipubic ramus
16. Site of attachment to perineal membrane
17. Deep fascia of penis
18. Superficial fascia of penis
19. Skin of penis
20. Prepuce (foreskin)
21. Glans

## Male Reproductive Organs

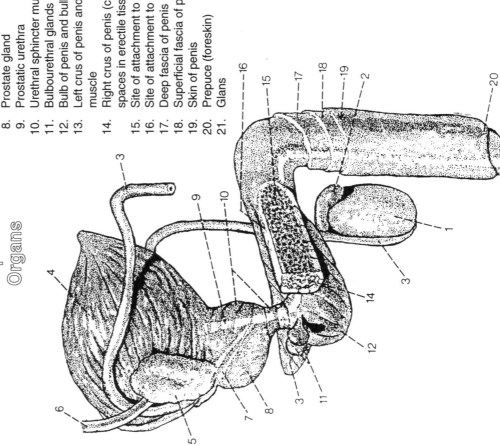

looking up
from below

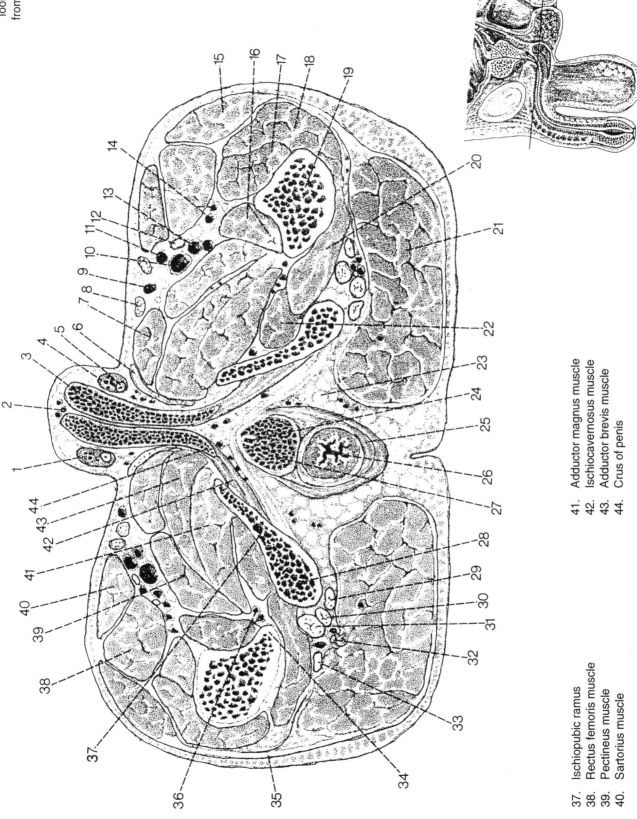

37. Ischiopubic ramus
38. Rectus femoris muscle
39. Pectineus muscle
40. Sartorius muscle

41. Adductor magnus muscle
42. Ischiocavernosus muscle
43. Adductor brevis muscle
44. Crus of penis

## Frontal Section of Male Pelvis

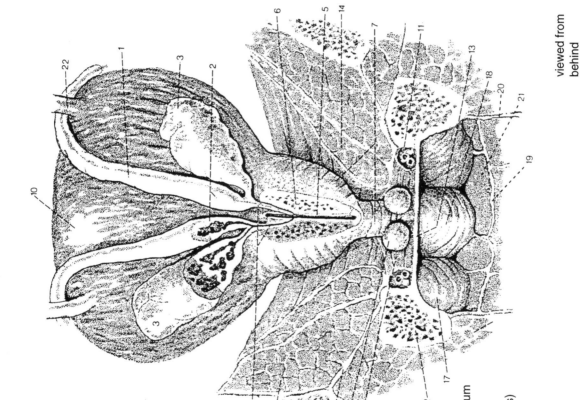

viewed from behind

*Color and label (at left):*

1. Ductus deferens
2. Ampulla of ductus deferens
3. Seminal vesicle
4. Ejaculatory duct
5. Urethra (prostatic part)
6. Prostate gland (wedge cut out)
7. Urethral sphincter muscle
8. Bulbourethral glands
9. Urethral sphicter muscle (lateral part)
10. Bladder
11. Pudendal canal, pudendal nerve, internal pudendal artery and vein
12. Ischiopubic ramus
13. Perineal membrane
14. Levator ani muscle (+ coccygeus muscle = pelvic diaphragm)
15. Obturator internus muscle
16. Obturator membrane
17. Ischiocavernosus muscle covering crus of penis
18. Bulbospongiosus muscle
19. Superficial perineal fascia (Colles' fascia)
20. Fascia lata (deep fascia of thigh)
21. Superficial perineal pouch (shown empty)
22. Ureter

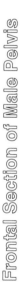

**SECTION 46**
**Penis, Testis Level**

*Color and label (below):*

1. Dartos muscle of scrotum
2. Epididymis
3. Cavity of tunica vaginalis
4. Right testis
5. Corpus cavernosus of the penis
6. Dorsal vessels of the penis
7. Urethra within the corpus spongiosum of penis
8. Testicular artery in spermatic cord (surrounded by pampiniform plexus)
9. Vas (ductus) deferens
10. Femoral artery
11. Femoral vein
12. Deep femoral artery and vein
13. Vastus medialis muscle
14. Lateral circumflex femoral vessels
15. Vastus intermedius muscle

*Continued...*

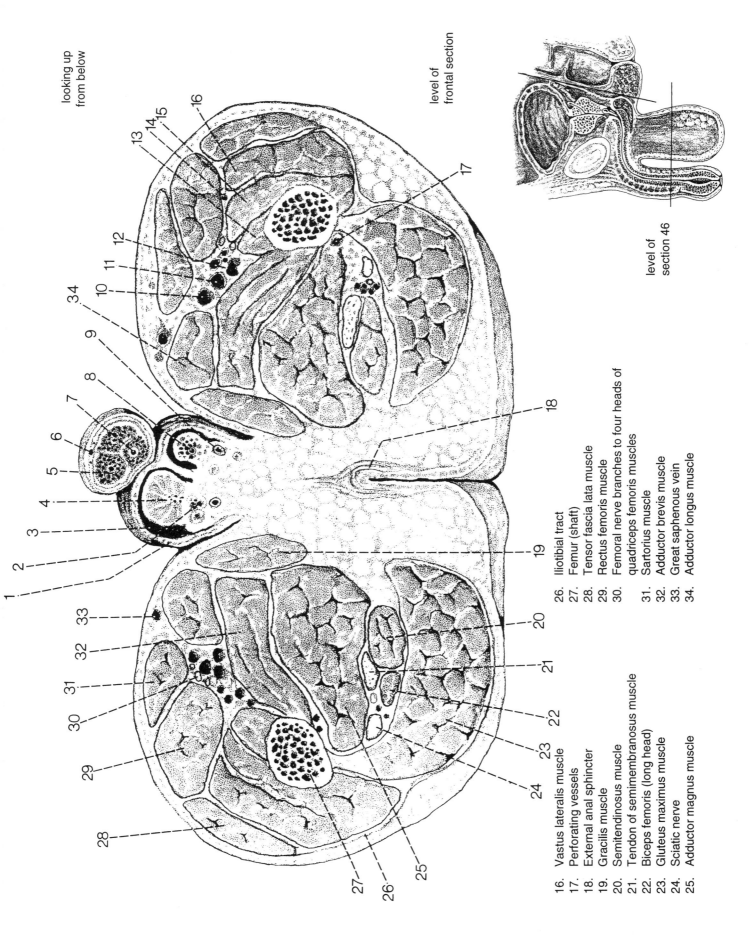

looking up
from below

level of
frontal section

level of
section 46

16. Vastus lateralis muscle
17. Perforating vessels
18. External anal sphincter
19. Gracilis muscle
20. Semitendinosus muscle
21. Tendon of semimembranosus muscle
22. Biceps femoris (long head)
23. Gluteus maximus muscle
24. Sciatic nerve
25. Adductor magnus muscle
26. Iliotibial tract
27. Femur (shaft)
28. Tensor fascia lata muscle
29. Rectus femoris muscle
30. Femoral nerve branches to four heads of
    quadriceps femoris muscles
31. Sartorius muscle
32. Adductor brevis muscle
33. Great saphenous vein
34. Adductor longus muscle

## Frontal Section of Male Pelvis

*Color and label (at left)*:

1. Perineal membrane
2. Urethra (membranous part)
3. Urethral sphincter muscle
4. Ejaculatory duct
5. Prostate gland
6. Ductus deferens (ampulla)
7. Seminal vesicle
8. Pelvic diaphragm
9. Obturator internus muscle
10. Inferior pubic ramus
11. Corpus cavernosus penis
12. Ischiocavernosus muscle
13. Corpus spongiosum penis
14. Bulbospongiosus muscle
15. Superifical perineal fascia (Colles')
16. Deep perineal fascia (Buck's)
17. Obturator membrane
18. Pudendal canal with internal
    pudendal artery, vein, and nerve
19. Fascia lata (deep fascia of thigh)
20. Ilium
21. Sheath of prostate gland
22. Transversalis fascia
23. Puboprostatic ligament

*after* Oelrich, TM: The urethral sphincter muscle in the male. American Journal of Anatomy 158:229–264, 1980.

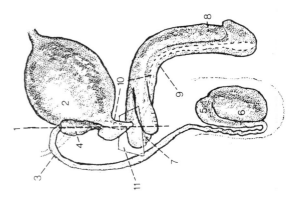

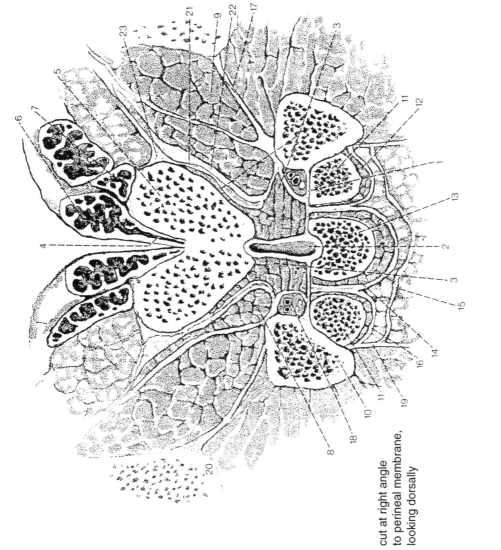

cut at right angle
to perineal membrane,
looking dorsally

*Color and label (at right)*:

1. Plane of frontal section
   shown above
2. Bladder
3. Ductus deferens
4. Seminal vesicle
5. Epididymis
6. Testis
7. Bulb of penis
8. Corpora cavernosa penis
9. Corpus spongiosum penis
10. Urethra
11. Perineal membrane
    (rendered transparent)

looking up
from below

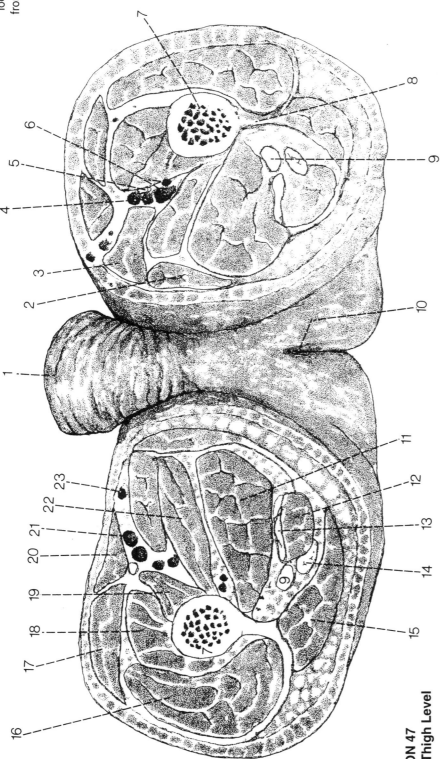

**SECTION 47**
**Upper Thigh Level**

*Color and label:*

1. Scrotum
2. Gracilis muscle
3. Adductor longus muscle
4. Femoral artery and vein
5. Saphenous nerve
6. Deep (profunda) femoral artery and vein
7. Femur (shaft)
8. Tendon of gluteus maximus muscle
9. Sciatic nerve
10. Anus
11. Adductor magnus muscle
12. Semitendinosus muscle

13. Tendon of semimembranosus muscle
14. Tendon of long head of biceps femoris muscle
15. Gluteus maximus muscle
16. Vastus lateralis muscle *
17. Rectus femoris muscle *
18. Vastus intermedius muscle *
19. Vastus medialis muscle *
20. Sartorius muscle
21. Femoral artery
22. Adductor brevis muscle
23. Great saphenous vein

* Part of quadriceps femoris.

# Pelvis – Female
## Sections 48 to 55

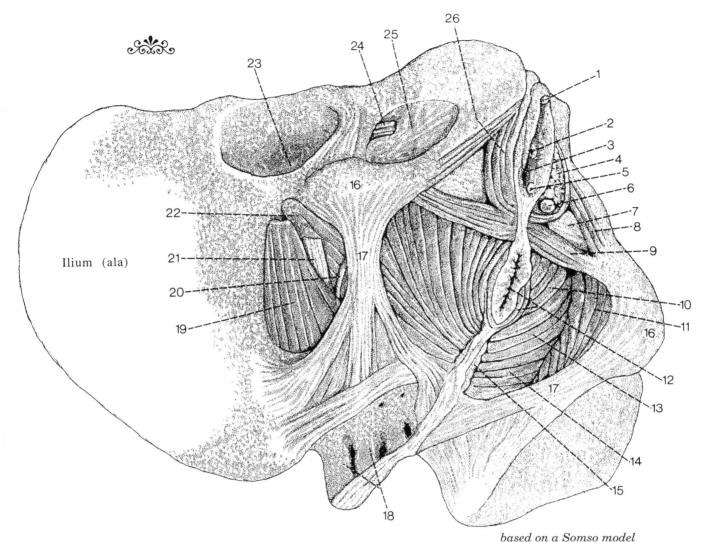

Ilium (ala)

based on a Somso model

*Color and label:*

1. Glans of clitoris
2. Opening of urethra
3. Vagina
4. Vestibular bulb (erectile tissue)
5. Opening of greater vestibular gland
6. Greater vestibular gland (Bartholin's)
7. Perineal membrane
8. Ischiocavernosus muscle—covers vestibular bulb (cut away on left side)
9. Superficial transverse perineus muscle
10. Puborectalis muscle
11. Obturator internus muscle
12. Anus and external sphincter muscle
13. Iliococcygeus muscle (part of levator ani muscle)
14. Coccygeus muscle (coccygeus + levator ani = pelvic diaphragm)
15. Coccyx
16. Ischial tuberosity
17. Sacrotuberous ligament
18. Sacrum (median crest)
19. Piriformis muscle
20. Pudendal nerve (accompanying internal pudendal artery and vein not shown)
21. Sciatic nerve
22. Obturator internus muscle (emerging from lesser sciatic foramen)
23. Acetabulum
24. Obturator nerve, artery, and vein
25. Obturator membrane
26. Bulbocavernosus muscle

# SECTION 48
## Ovaries, Fundus of Uterus Level

*Color and label (below):*

1. Linea alba
2. Ileum
3. Sigmoid colon
4. Oviduct (fimbria)
5. External iliac vein
6. External iliac artery
7. Femoral nerve
8. Pudendal nerve
9. Inferior gluteal nerve, artery, and vein
10. Fundus of uterus
11. Rectum
12. Sacrum
13. Ovary
14. Sciatic nerve
15. Gluteus maximus muscle
16. Obturator nerve and artery
17. Ilium
18. Gluteus medius muscle
19. Superior gluteal artery and vein
20. Gluteus minimus muscle
21. Tensor fascia lata muscle
22. Sartorius muscle
23. Iliopsoas muscle
24. Internal abdominal oblique muscle
25. Transversus abdominis muscle
26. Ureter
27. Inferior epigastric artery and vein
28. Rectus abdominis muscle

*Color and label (at left):*

1. Uterus (body)
2. Cervix of uterus
3. Vagina
4. Rectouterine pouch (of Douglas)
5. Bladder
6. Urethra
7. Anus
8. Rectum
9. Round ligament of uterus
10. Transverse vesical fold
11. Uterine tube (ampulla)
12. Ovary
13. Fimbriae (fimbria)
14. Infundibulum
15. Suspensory ligament of the ovary
16. Vesicouterine pouch
17. Posterior lip of uterus
18. Glans of clitoris and prepuce
19. Pubic symphysis
20. Posterior fornix of vagina

## Female Pelvis, Median Section

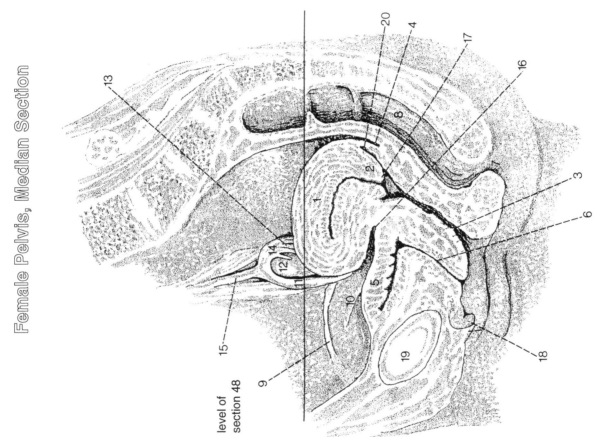

level of
section 48

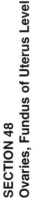

looking up
from below

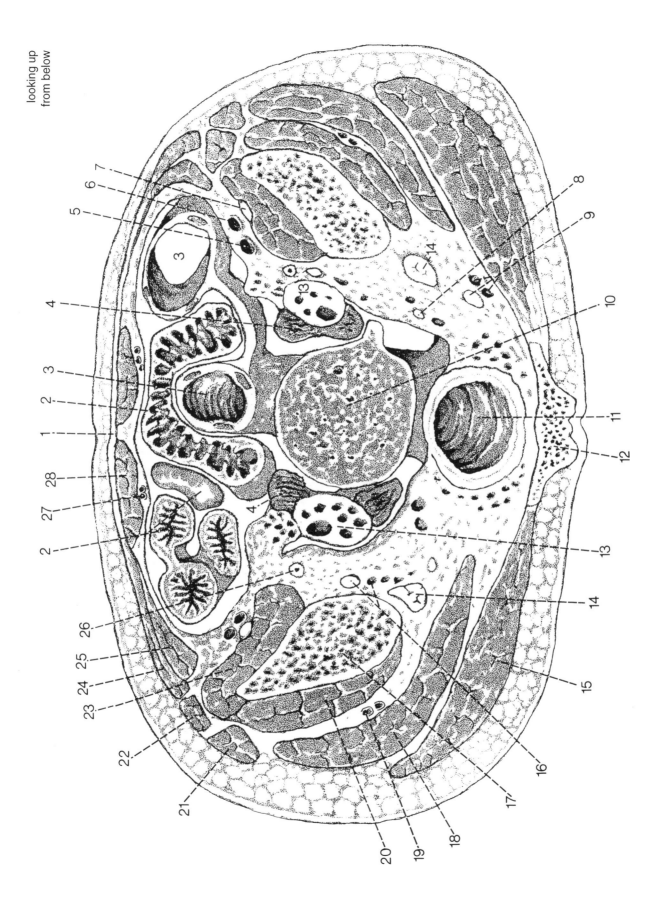

## Uterus and Related Structures

*Color and label (at left)\*:*

1. Fundus of uterus
2. Cavity of uterus
3. Body of uterus
4. Cervix of uterus—supravaginal part
5. Cervix of uterus—vaginal part
6. Cervical canal
7. Vagina
8. Opening of uterus
9. Anterior lip of cervix
10. Lateral fornices of vagina
11. Isthmus of uterus
12. Endometrium (mucosal lining)
13. Myometrium (smooth muscle)
14. Perimetrium (peritoneum, tunica serosa)
15. Broad ligament of uterus (mesometrium)
16. Mesovarium (broad ligament)
17. Mesosalpinx (broad ligament)
18. Uterine tube
19. Infundibulum (of uterine tube)
20. Ampulla (of uterine tube)
21. Fimbriae (of uterine tube)
22. Ureter
23. Uterine artery
24. Rectouterine (ureterosacral) ligament
25. Lateral cervical ligament (cardial ligament, Mackenrodt's ligament)
26. Ovary
27. Proper ligament of ovary
28. Ovarian artery

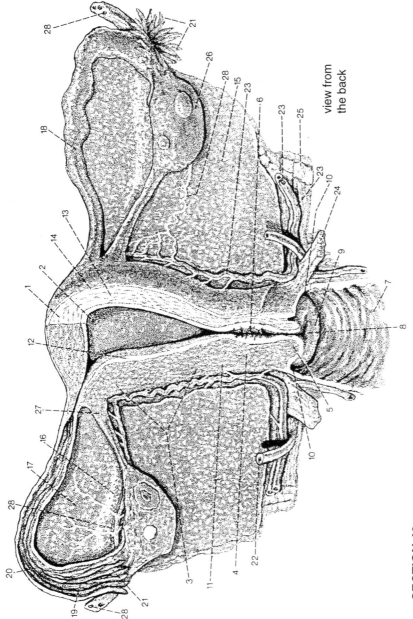

view from the back

**SECTION 49**
**Uterus, Broad Ligament Level**

*Color and label (below):*

1. Femoral nerve
2. External iliac artery
3. External iliac vein
4. Ileum
5. Mesentery of small intestine
6. Rectus abdominis muscles
7. Inferior epigastric artery and vein (often divide into two or more collateral branches)
8. Obturator nerve and vein (artery often arises from external iliac artery)

9. Sigmoid colon (so named because it resembles the Greek letter sigma
10. Transversus abdominis muscle
11. Internal abdominal oblique muscle
12. Iliopsoas muscle (formed by union of psoas major and iliacus muscles)
13. Sartorius muscle

*Continued...*

looking up
from below

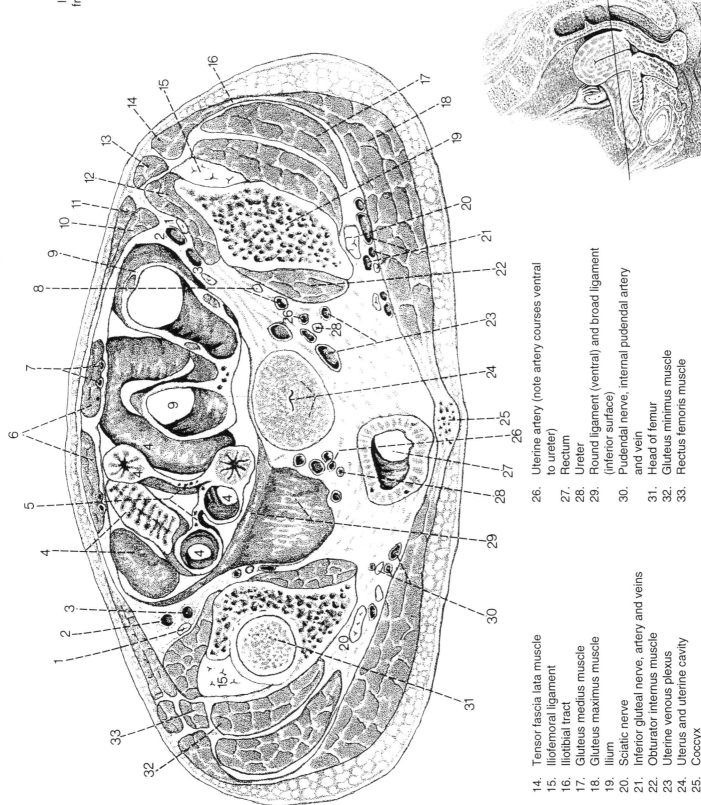

14. Tensor fascia lata muscle
15. Iliofemoral ligament
16. Iliotibial tract
17. Gluteus medius muscle
18. Gluteus maximus muscle
19. Ilium
20. Sciatic nerve
21. Inferior gluteal nerve, artery and veins
22. Obturator internus muscle
23. Uterine venous plexus
24. Uterus and uterine cavity
25. Coccyx

26. Uterine artery (note artery courses ventral to ureter)
27. Rectum
28. Ureter
29. Round ligament (ventral) and broad ligament (inferior surface)
30. Pudendal nerve, internal pudendal artery and vein
31. Head of femur
32. Gluteus minimus muscle
33. Rectus femoris muscle

## Female Pelvis, Front and Above View

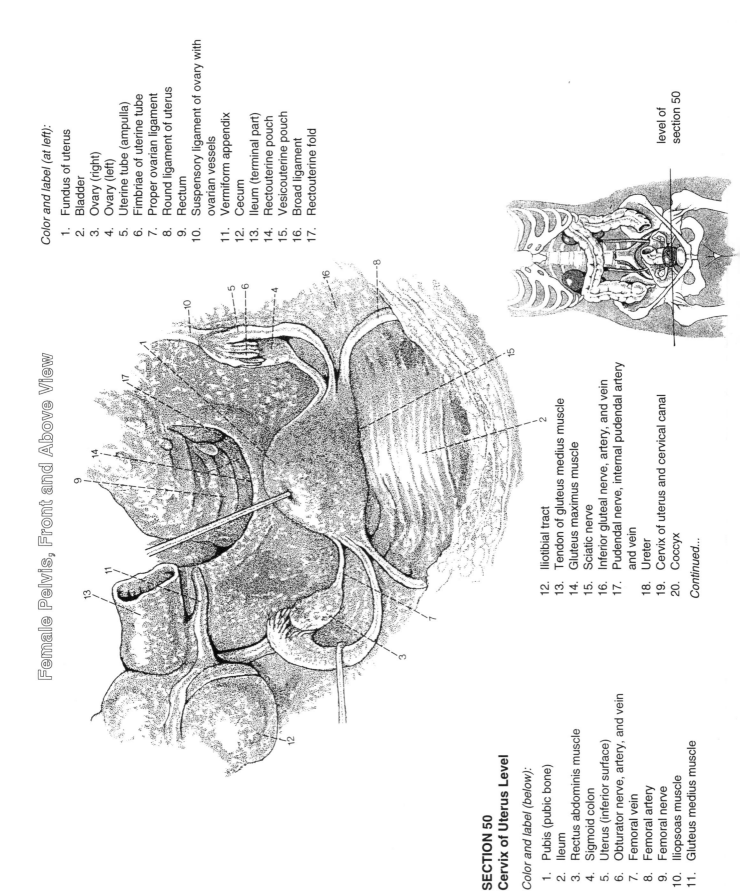

level of
section 50

Continued...

Color and label (at left):

1. Fundus of uterus
2. Bladder
3. Ovary (right)
4. Ovary (left)
5. Uterine tube (ampulla)
6. Fimbriae of uterine tube
7. Proper ovarian ligament
8. Round ligament of uterus
9. Rectum
10. Suspensory ligament of ovary with ovarian vessels
11. Vermiform appendix
12. Cecum
13. Ileum (terminal part)
14. Rectouterine pouch
15. Vesicouterine pouch
16. Broad ligament
17. Rectouterine fold

## SECTION 50
### Cervix of Uterus Level

Color and label (below):

1. Pubis (pubic bone)
2. Ileum
3. Rectus abdominis muscle
4. Sigmoid colon
5. Uterus (inferior surface)
6. Obturator nerve, artery, and vein
7. Femoral vein
8. Femoral artery
9. Femoral nerve
10. Iliopsoas muscle
11. Gluteus medius muscle

12. Iliotibial tract
13. Tendon of gluteus medius muscle
14. Gluteus maximus muscle
15. Sciatic nerve
16. Inferior gluteal nerve, artery, and vein
17. Pudendal nerve, internal pudendal artery and vein
18. Ureter
19. Cervix of uterus and cervical canal
20. Coccyx

looking up
from below

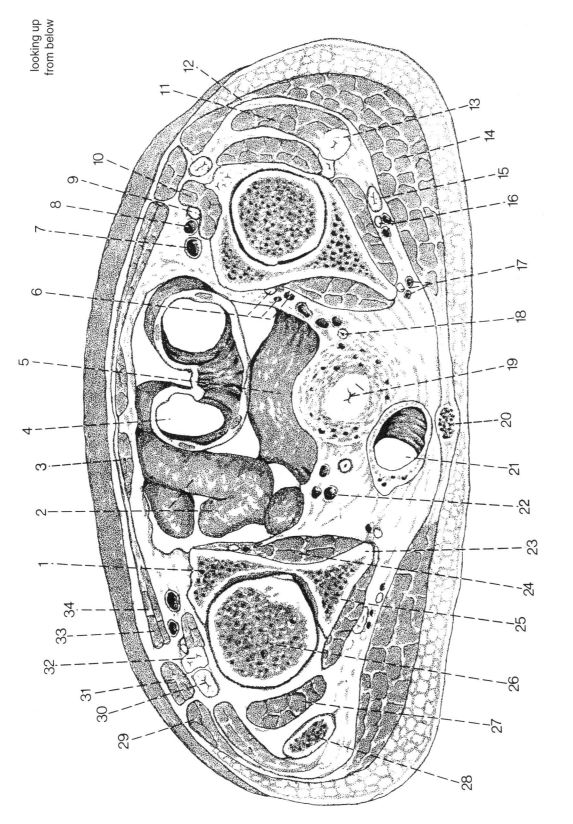

21. Rectum
22. Uterine venous plexus in uterosacral ligament
23. Spine of ischium
24. Obturator internus muscle
25. Ischium
26. Head of femur
27. Gluteus minimus muscle

28. Greater trochanter of femur
29. Tensor fascia lata muscle
30. Rectus femoris tendon
31. Sartorius muscle
32. Tendon of iliopsoas muscle and femoral nerve
33. Internal abdominal oblique muscle
34. Transversus abdominis muscle

## Uterus

**SECTION 51**
**Vagina, Head of Femur Level**

*Color and label (below):*

1. Head of femur
2. Femoral nerve (branches)
3. Femoral artery
4. Femoral vein
5. Pubis
6. Ileum of small intestine
7. Rectus abdominis muscle
8. Obturator nerve, artery, and vein
9. Ligament of head of femur
10. Lip of acetabulum (Lat., labrum acetabulare)
11. Sartorius muscle
12. Iliofemoral ligament
13. Tensor fascia lata muscle
14. Gluteus minimus muscle
15. Gluteus medius muscle
16. Ischiofemoral ligament
17. Gluteus maximus muscle
18. Inferior gluteal artery and vein
19. Sacrotuberous ligament
20. Pudendal nerve, internal pudendal artery and vein
21. Vaginal venous plexus
22. Vagina
23. Rectum
24. Levator ani muscle
25. Inferior rectal nerve
26. Ureter
27. Obturator internus muscle
28. Ischial tuberosity
29. Sciatic nerve
30. Gemellus superior muscle
31. Greater trochanter of femur
32. Iliotibial tract
33. Rectus femoris muscle (partly tendinous)
34. Neck of femur (usually a "broken hip" is a broken femoral neck)

*Color and label (at left):*

1. Fundus of uterus
2. Uterus (body)
3. Cervix of uterus (vaginal part)
4. Ovary
5. Suspensory ligament of ovary with ovarian artery and vein (cut)
6. Uterine, or fallopian, tube (also oviduct, or salpinx—Gr., trumpet or tube)
7. Infundibulum of uterine tube
8. Fimbria of uterine tube
9. Round ligament of uterus
10. Mesosalpinx (part of broad ligament attached to uterine tube)
11. Mesovarium (part of broad ligament attached to ovary)
12. Mesometrium (part of broad ligament attached to uterus)
13. Posterior fornix of vagina
14. Lateral cervical ligament (cardinal ligament or Mackenrodt's ligament) and uterine vessels
15. Vagina (cut, showing rugae)
16. Rectum (cut)
17. Uterosacral ligament and fold

viewed from the left

looking up
from below

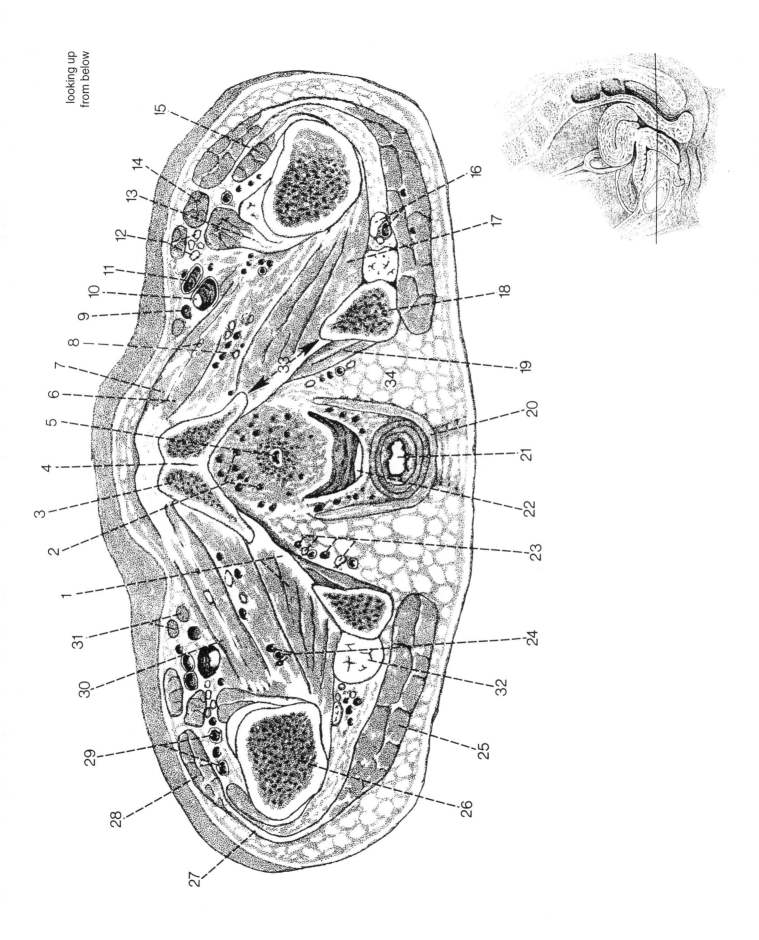

## Blood Supply of Female Pelvis

**SECTION 52**
**Bladder, Vagina Level**

*Color and label (below):*

1. Femur
2. Neck of femur
3. Iliopsoas muscle and tendon
4. Femoral artery
5. Femoral vein
6. Obturator externus muscle
7. Obturator nerve, anterior division
8. Bladder (cut above urethra, inside of superior wall visible through opening)
9. Interpubic disk and cavity of pubic symphysis
10. Pubis (body)
11. Bladder, inferior surface
12. Pectineus muscle
13. Obturator membrane
14. Femoral nerve (branches)
15. Iliofemoral ligament
16. Tensor fascia lata muscle
17. Iliotibial tract
18. Quadratus femoris muscle
19. Sciatic nerve
20. Inferior gluteal artery and vein, posterior cutaneous nerve of thigh
21. Common tendon of origin of hamstring muscles
22. Obturator nerve (divided) and vein
23. Ischiorectal fat pad within ischiorectal fossa
24. Levator ani muscle, puborectalis part
25. Rectum
26. Vagina
27. Venous plexus of bladder
28. Obturator internus muscle
29. Ischial tuberosity
30. Obturator nerve (posterior division), obturator vessels
31. Gluteus maximus muscle

*Color and label (at left):*

1. Aorta
2. Inferior mesenteric artery
3. Right common iliac artery
4. Right external iliac artery and vein
5. Left common iliac artery and vein
6. Left external iliac artery and vein (cut)
7. Internal iliac artery
8. Superior gluteal artery
9. Inferior gluteal artery
10. Internal pudendal artery
11. Inferior rectal artery
12. Obturator artery
13. Umbilical artery
14. Superior vesical artery
15. Obliterated part of umbilical artery (medial umbilical fold)
16. Uterine artery
17. Vaginal artery
18. Piriformis muscle
19. Coccygeus muscle
20. Levator ani muscle
21. Obturator internus muscle
22. External anal sphincter
23. Labia minora
24. Glans of clitoris
25. Ureter
26. Uterus
27. Bladder

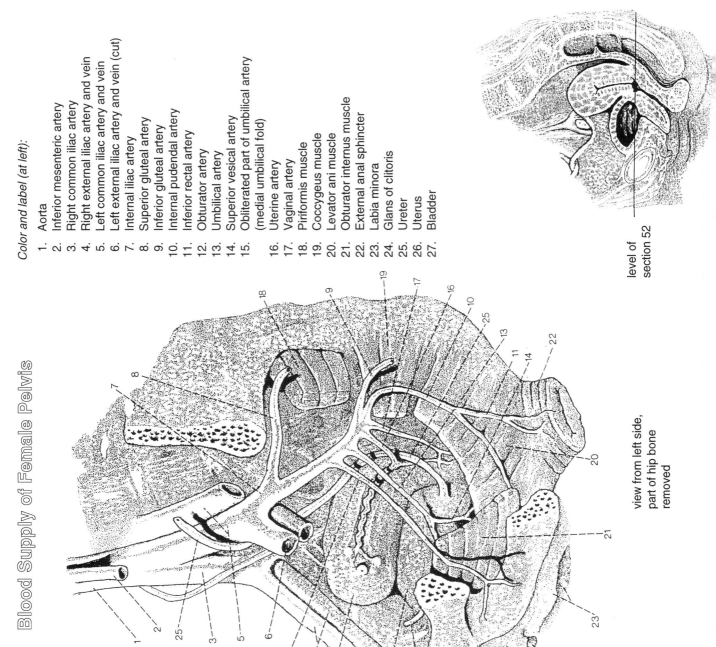

view from left side, part of hip bone removed

level of section 52

looking up
from below

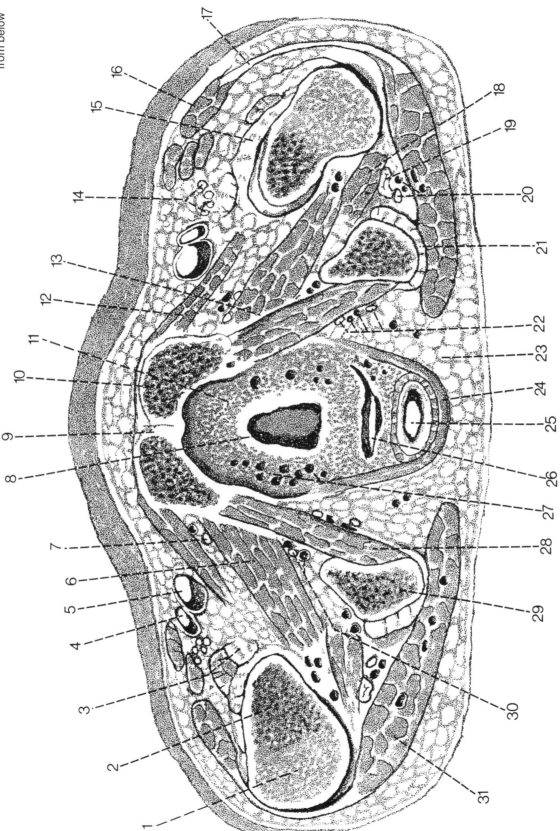

Female Urogenital Sphincter

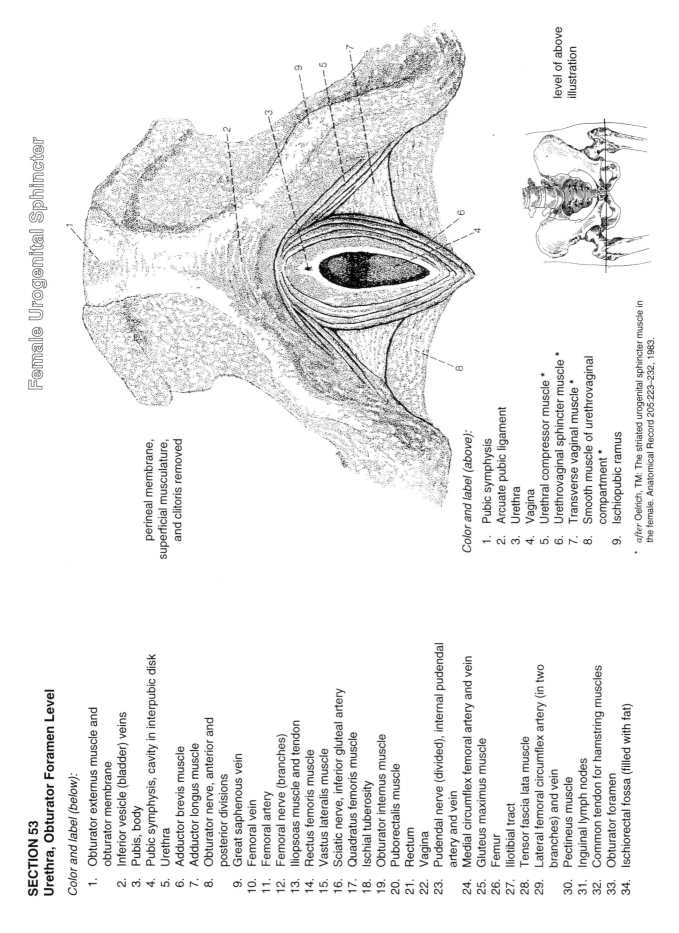

level of above
illustration

perineal membrane,
superficial musculature,
and clitoris removed

**SECTION 53**
**Urethra, Obturator Foramen Level**

*Color and label (below):*

1. Obturator externus muscle and
   obturator membrane
2. Inferior vesicle (bladder) veins
3. Pubis, body
4. Pubic symphysis, cavity in interpubic disk
5. Urethra
6. Adductor brevis muscle
7. Adductor longus muscle
8. Obturator nerve, anterior and
   posterior divisions
9. Great saphenous vein
10. Femoral vein
11. Femoral artery
12. Femoral nerve (branches)
13. Iliopsoas muscle and tendon
14. Rectus femoris muscle
15. Vastus lateralis muscle
16. Sciatic nerve, inferior gluteal artery
17. Quadratus femoris muscle
18. Ischial tuberosity
19. Obturator internus muscle
20. Puborectalis muscle
21. Rectum
22. Vagina
23. Pudendal nerve (divided), internal pudendal
    artery and vein
24. Medial circumflex femoral artery and vein
25. Gluteus maximus muscle
26. Femur
27. Iliotibial tract
28. Tensor fascia lata muscle
29. Lateral femoral circumflex artery (in two
    branches) and vein
30. Pectineus muscle
31. Inguinal lymph nodes
32. Common tendon for hamstring muscles
33. Obturator foramen
34. Ischiorectal fossa (filled with fat)

*Color and label (above):*

1. Pubic symphysis
2. Arcuate pubic ligament
3. Urethra
4. Vagina
5. Urethral compressor muscle *
6. Urethrovaginal sphincter muscle *
7. Transverse vaginal muscle *
8. Smooth muscle of urethrovaginal
   compartment *
9. Ischiopubic ramus

\* *after* Oelrich, TM: The striated urogenital sphincter muscle in
the female. Anatomical Record 205:223–232, 1983.

looking up
from below

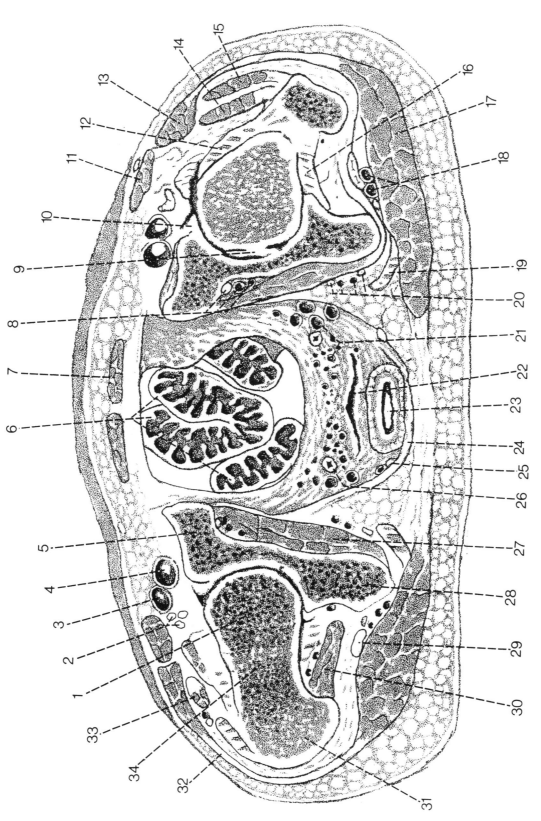

## Female Erectile Tissue

### SECTION 54
### Clitoris, Vagina Level

*Color and label (below):*

1. Ischiopubic ramus
2. Mons pubis
3. Crus of clitoris
4. Body of clitoris
5. Urethra
6. Adductor longus muscle
7. Adductor brevis muscle
8. External pudendal vein (tributary of great saphenous vein)
9. Femoral vein
10. Femoral artery
11. Profunda femoris (deep femoral) artery and vein
12. Tendon of iliopsoas muscle with iliofemoral ligament
13. Vastus lateralis muscle
14. Iliotibial tract
15. Femur
16. Lesser trochanter of femur
17. Obturator internus muscle
18. Vaginal venous plexus
19. Recto-anal junction
20. Puborectalis muscle (part of levator ani)
21. Vagina
22. Perineal nerve (branch of pudendal nerve) and vessels
23. Common tendon of origin of hamstring muscles
24. Adductor magnus
25. Sciatic nerve
26. Gluteus maximus muscle
27. Tensor fascia lata muscle
28. Branches of femoral nerve
29. Pectineus muscle
30. Anterior and posterior divisions of obturator nerve
31. Great saphenous vein

*Color and label (at left):*

1. Suspensory ligament of clitoris
2. Body of clitoris *
3. Glans of clitoris
4. Vestibular bulb **
5. Commissure of vestibular bulb (joins the two vestibular bulbs to underside of clitoris)
6. Left crus of clitoris
7. Greater vestibular gland and duct—secretes lubricating mucus (Bartholin's gland)
8. External urethral orifice
9. Labium minus (cut)
10. Orifice of greater vestibular glands

\* Clitoris is richly supplied with nerves and its stimulation plays a dominant role in sexual response.

\*\* Clitoris and vestibular bulb consist of erectile tissue and become tumescent during sexual arousal.

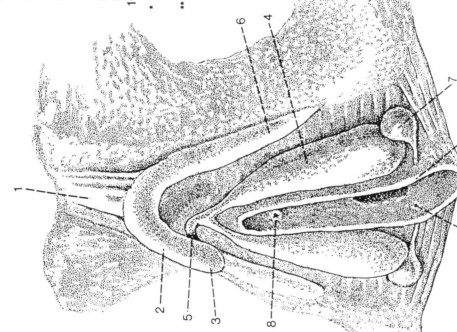

looking up
from below

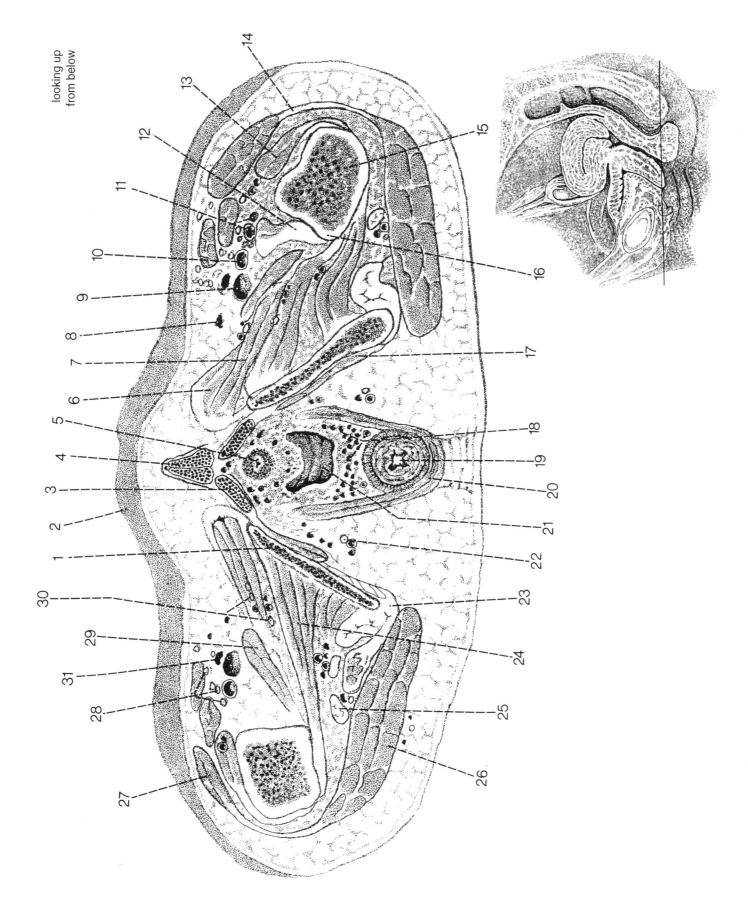

## SECTION 55
## Vestibular Bulb, Greater Vestibular Gland, Upper Thigh Level

*Color and label (below):*

1. Clitoris (glans)
2. Prepuce of clitoris
3. Vestibule of vagina (common opening for vagina and urethra)
4. Urethra (external orifice)
5. Vestibular bulb (erectile tissue)
6. Gracilis muscle
7. Tributary of great saphenous vein
8. Great saphenous vein
9. Femoral vein
10. Femoral artery
11. Pectineus muscle
12. Vastus intermedius muscle
13. Lateral circumflex femoral artery
14. Vastus lateralis muscle
15. Femur
16. Sciatic nerve
17. Tendon of long head of biceps femoris muscle
18. Tendon of semimembranosus muscle
19. Ischiorectal fossa
20. Anus
21. Posterior labial venous plexus
22. Greater vestibular gland (Bartholin's)
23. Adductor magnus (two parts)
24. Semitendinosus muscle, tendons of biceps femoris (long head) and semimembranosus muscles
25. Gluteus maximus muscle
26. Iliotibial tract
27. Tensor fascia lata muscle
28. Rectus femoris muscle
29. Branches of femoral nerve
30. Obturator nerve (anterior branch) and obturator vessels
31. Adductor brevis muscle
32. Obturator nerve (posterior branch) and vessels
33. Adductor longus muscle

Female Perineum

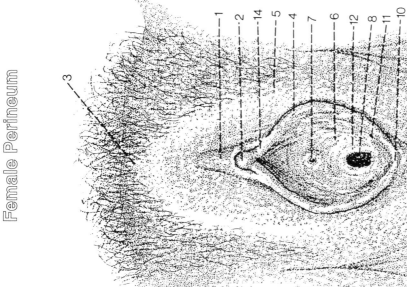

*Color and label (at left):*

1. Prepuce of clitoris
2. Glans of clitoris
3. Mons pubis
4. Labium minus pudendi
5. Labium majus pudendi
6. Vestibule of vagina
7. External urethral ostium
8. Ostium of vagina
9. Posterior labial commissure
10. Frenulum of labia minora (Forchet)
11. Opening of greater vestibular glands
12. Hymen
13. Anus
14. Frenulum of clitoris

looking up
from below

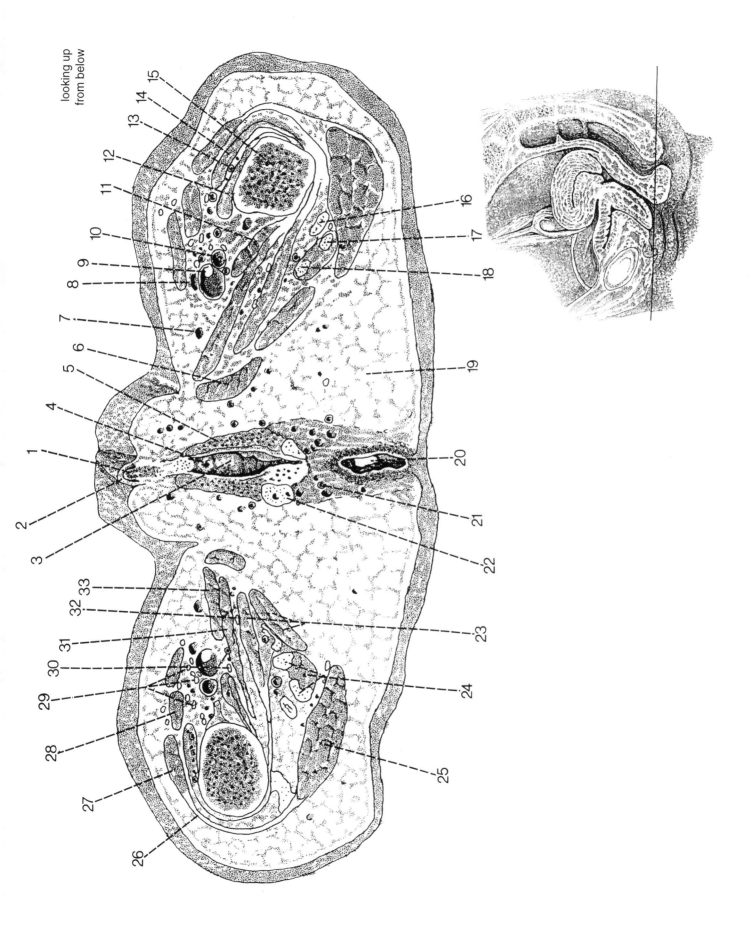

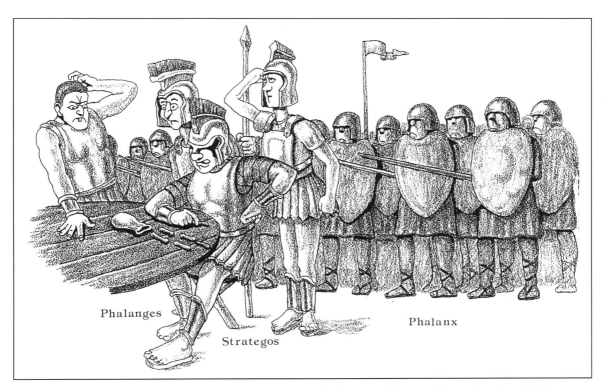

Phalanges

Phalanx

Strategos

**The *phalanx* (Gr.) was a compact formation of infantry soldiers** with overlapping shields and projecting spears. It was developed by Philip II of Macedon and later used extensively by Alexander the Great.

The *phalanges* (pl. of phalanx) are the bones of the fingers and toes. Supposedly it was Aristotle who gave them this name. He thought that the bones within the fingers resembled a formation of infantry phalanges drawn up for battle. The thumb (Lat., *pollex*) has only two phalanges, as does the big toe (Lat., *hallux*). Each finger has three phalanges. Thus, each hand and each foot has fourteen phalanges (2+3+3+3+3 = 14). The wrist (Lat., *carpus*) consists of eight carpal bones in two rows of four. Within the palm of the hand are the five metacarpal (beyond the carpus) bones. These are the largest and strongest bones of the hand, especially the second and third metacarpal bones which directly receive the force of impact when the fist strikes a blow.

The foot has seven tarsal bones, five metatarsal bones, and fourteen phalanges (Gr., *tarsos*—flat surface, sole of the foot, edge of the eyelid). In anatomy, "tarsus" refers specifically to the instep of the foot or to that part of the foot containing the seven tarsal bones.

A Greek general was a *strategos*; hence our word "strategy" (Gr., *stratos*—"army" + *agein*—"to lead" = *strategein* which was shortened to strategos.

In the cartoon above, the general and his entourage were drawn by my former student Wayne Timmerman. I added the troops forming a phalanx.

# Muscles of Anterior Thigh

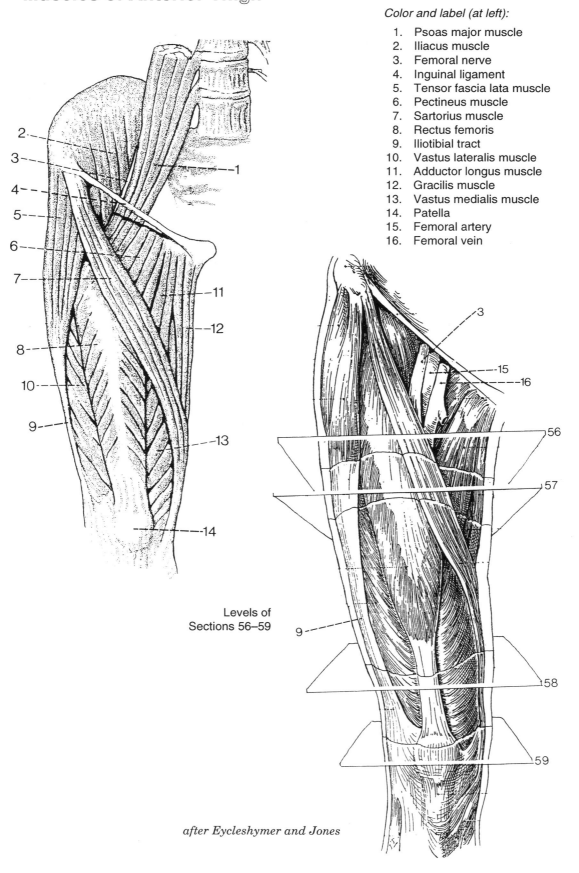

Color and label (at left):

1. Psoas major muscle
2. Iliacus muscle
3. Femoral nerve
4. Inguinal ligament
5. Tensor fascia lata muscle
6. Pectineus muscle
7. Sartorius muscle
8. Rectus femoris
9. Iliotibial tract
10. Vastus lateralis muscle
11. Adductor longus muscle
12. Gracilis muscle
13. Vastus medialis muscle
14. Patella
15. Femoral artery
16. Femoral vein

Levels of
Sections 56–59

*after Eycleshymer and Jones*

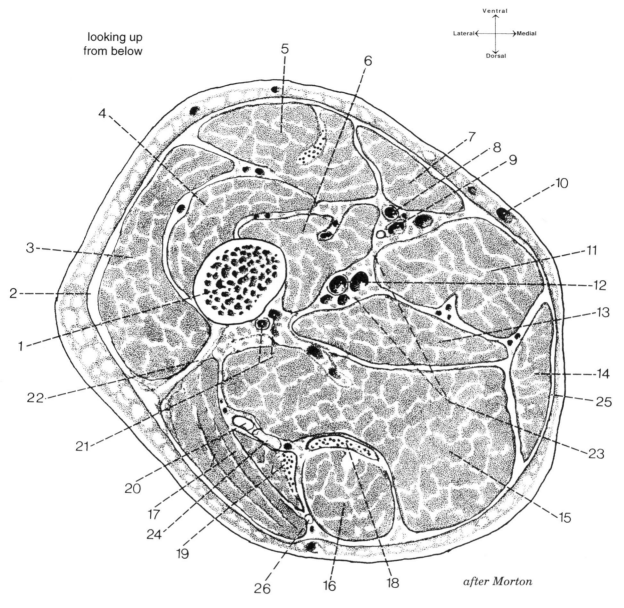

looking up
from below

Ventral
Lateral← →Medial
Dorsal

*after Morton*

## SECTION 56
## Right Upper Thigh*

*Color and label:*

1. Femur (shaft)
2. Iliotibial tract (thickened part of fascia lata)
3. Vastus lateralis muscle
4. Vastus intermedius muscle
5. Rectus femoris muscle
6. Vastus medialis
7. Sartorius muscle
8. Femoral artery
9. Femoral vein
10. Great saphenous vein
11. Adductor longus muscle
12. Profunda (deep) femoris artery and vein
13. Adductor brevis muscle
14. Gracilis muscle
15. Adductor magnus muscle

16. Semitendinosus muscle
17. Gluteus maximus muscle
18. Semimembranosus tendon
19. Biceps femoris muscle(long head)
20. Common peroneal nerve
21. Perforating artery and vein
22. Lateral intermuscular septum
23. Medial intermuscular septum
24. Tibial nerve
25. Fascia lata (deep fascia of thigh)
26. Posterior femoral cutaneous nerve

* In anatomy the region of the lower limb above the knee is
   designated "thigh". The term "leg" is reserved for that
   region below the knee and above the ankle.

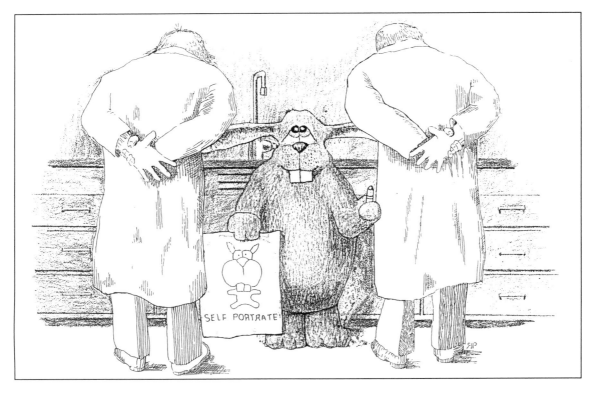

**The term *somesthesia* combines two Greek words**: *soma*—"body" or "corpus" (as opposed to the *psyche* or "mind") + *aisthesis*—"sensation." Hence, "bodily sensation" or "consciousness of the body." This rabbit was asked to draw his self-portrait. The obvious distortion, with the head and snout being much too large for the body and limbs, is the result of the head and snout having a disproportionately large cerebral cortical representation compared to that of the remainder of the body.

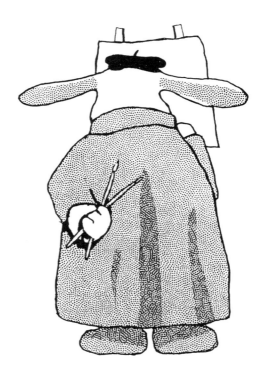

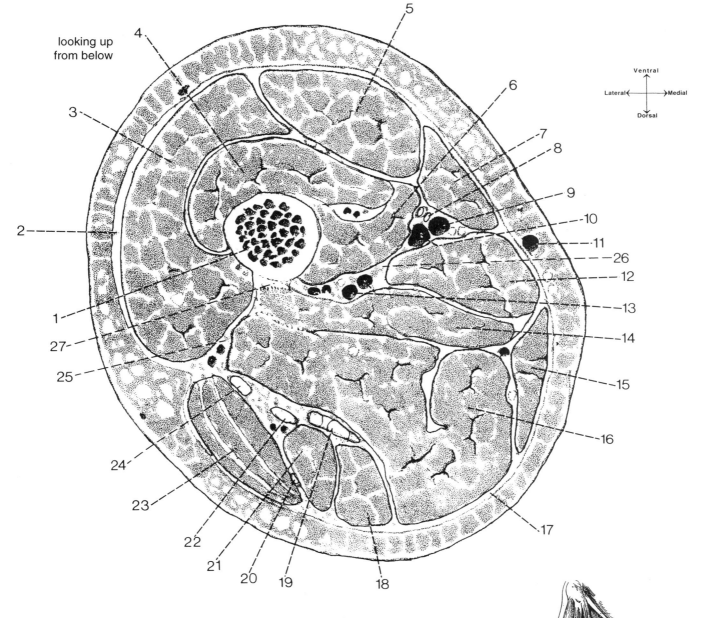

looking up
from below

Ventral
Lateral ← → Medial
Dorsal

*after Morton*

**SECTION 57**
**Right Middle Thigh**

*Color and label:*

1. Femur (shaft)
2. Iliotibial tract (thickened portion of fascia lata)
3. Vastus lateralis muscle
4. Vastus intermedialis muscle
5. Rectus femoris muscle
6. Vastus medialis
7. Sartorius muscle
8. Saphenous nerve (terminal cutaneous branch of femoral nerve)
9. Femoral artery
10. Femoral vein
11. Great saphenous vein
12. Adductor longus muscle
13. Profunda (deep) femoral artery and vein

14. Adductor brevis muscle
15. Gracilis muscle
16. Adductor magnus muscle
17. Fascia lata (deep fascia of thigh)
18. Semitendinosus muscle
19. Tendon of semimembranosus muscle
20. Posterior femoral cutaneous nerve
21. Long head of biceps femoris muscle
22. Tibial nerve
23. Gluteus maximus muscle
24. Common peroneal nerve
25. Lateral intermuscular septum
26. Medial intermuscular septum
27. Linea aspera (Lat., rough line)

# Muscles of Buttock and Posterior Thigh

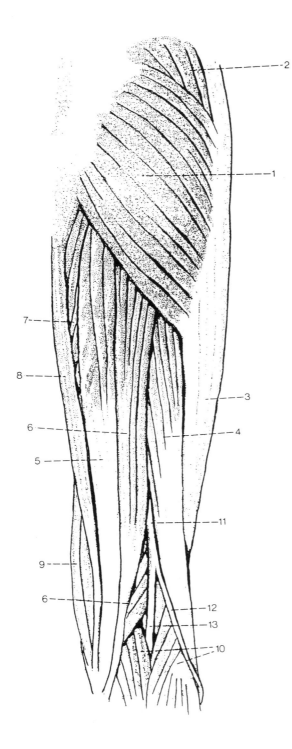

*Color and label (at left):*

1. Gluteus maximus
2. Gluteus medius
3. Iliotibial tract
4. Biceps femoris
5. Semitendinosus
6. Semimembranosus
7. Adductor magnus (posterior vertical part)
8. Gracilis
9. Sartorius
10. Medial and lateral heads of gastrocnemius
11. Sciatic nerve
12. Common peroneal nerve
13. Tibial nerve

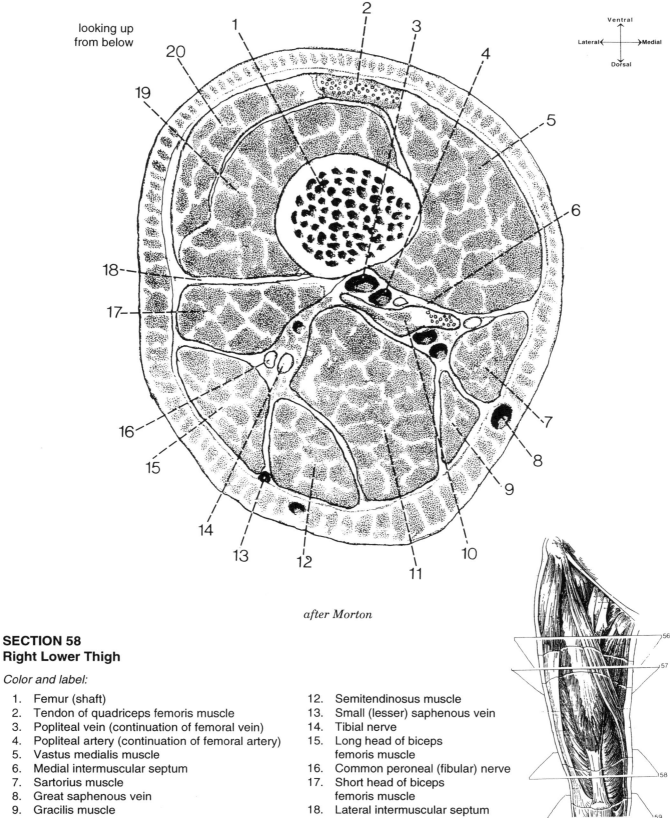

looking up
from below

Ventral
Lateral← →Medial
Dorsal

*after Morton*

## SECTION 58
## Right Lower Thigh

*Color and label:*

1. Femur (shaft)
2. Tendon of quadriceps femoris muscle
3. Popliteal vein (continuation of femoral vein)
4. Popliteal artery (continuation of femoral artery)
5. Vastus medialis muscle
6. Medial intermuscular septum
7. Sartorius muscle
8. Great saphenous vein
9. Gracilis muscle
10. Adductor magnus muscle and tendon
11. Semimembranosus muscle
12. Semitendinosus muscle
13. Small (lesser) saphenous vein
14. Tibial nerve
15. Long head of biceps femoris muscle
16. Common peroneal (fibular) nerve
17. Short head of biceps femoris muscle
18. Lateral intermuscular septum
19. Vastus intermedius muscle
20. Vastus lateralis muscle

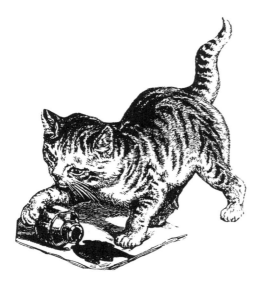

**If you love cats, you are an *ail-
urophile*** (Gr., *ailouros*—"cat" +
*phile*—"lover" or "one having an
affinity for" or "strong attraction to").
If you have a fear or hatred of cats,
you are an *ailurophobe* (*ailuoros*—
"cat" + *phobos*—"fear"). Of course,
if your cat has just ruined your life's
work, then you could be expected to
be a little upset with your feline com-
panion.

A possible explanation as to why men
have a prominent superciliary arch,
whereas women do not, is that men
frown more and thus have more highly developed corrugator supercilium
muscles. Frowning on the part of men
is most likely due to their trying to
figure out what makes women tick.

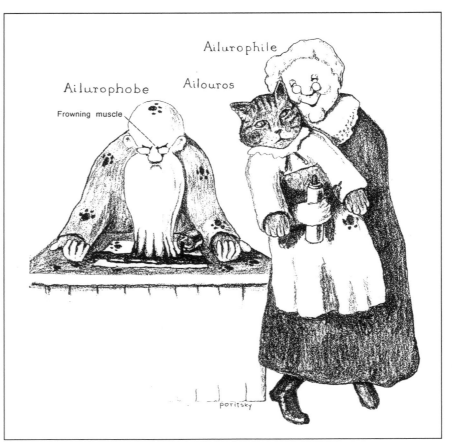

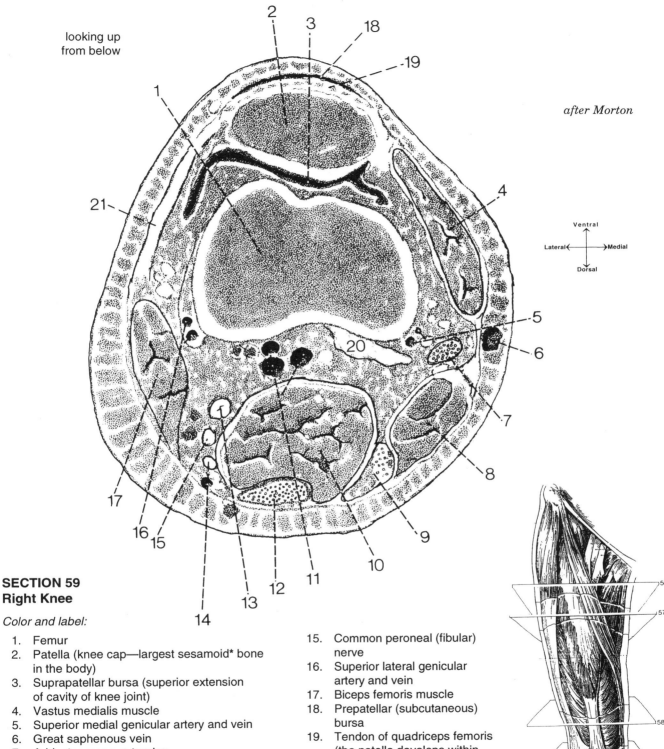

looking up
from below

after Morton

Ventral
Lateral ← → Medial
Dorsal

20

**SECTION 59**
**Right Knee**

*Color and label:*

1. Femur
2. Patella (knee cap—largest sesamoid* bone in the body)
3. Suprapatellar bursa (superior extension of cavity of knee joint)
4. Vastus medialis muscle
5. Superior medial genicular artery and vein
6. Great saphenous vein
7. Adductor magnus tendon
8. Sartorius muscle
9. Gracilis muscle and tendon
10. Semimembranosus muscle
11. Popliteal vein (divided) and artery
12. Semitendinosus tendon
13. Tibial nerve
14. Lateral sural cutaneous nerve

15. Common peroneal (fibular) nerve
16. Superior lateral genicular artery and vein
17. Biceps femoris muscle
18. Prepatellar (subcutaneous) bursa
19. Tendon of quadriceps femoris (the patella develops within the quadriceps tendon)
20. Tendinous origin of medial head of gastrocnemius muscle
21. Iliotibial tract

* Sesamoid bones are found in tendons. Their name comes from their supposed resemblance to sesame seeds.

Lower Extremity

Right Leg

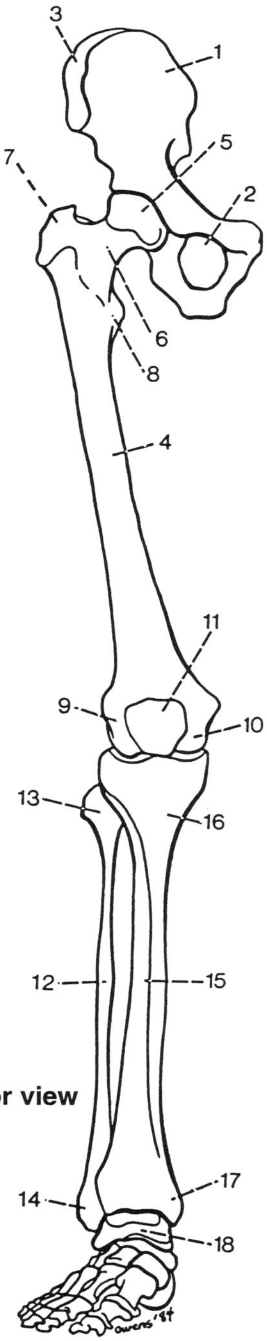

*Color and label (at left):*
1. Coxal bone (hip bone)
2. Obturator foramen
3. Iliac crest
4. Femur
5. Head of femur
6. Neck of femur
7. Greater trochanter
8. Lesser trochanter
9. Lateral epicondyle
10. Medial epicondyle
11. Patella
12. Fibula
13. Head of fibula
14. Lateral malleolus
15. Tibia
16. Tibial tuberosity
17. Medial malleolus
18. Talus

*Color and label (at right):*
1. Ischial tuberosity
2. Greater trochanter
3. Lesser trochanter
4. Intertrochanteric crest
5. Linea aspera
6. Adductor tubercle
7. Medial condyle
8. Lateral condyle
9. Tibia
10. Fibula
11. Talus
12. Calcaneus

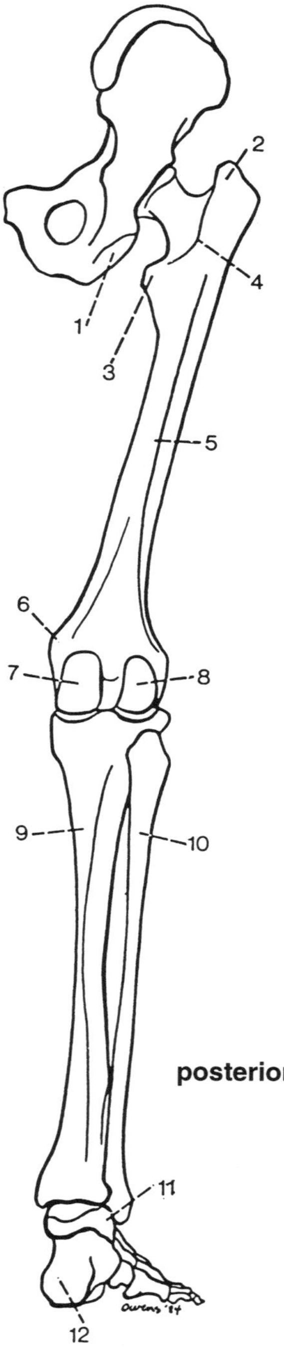

**anterior view**

**posterior view**

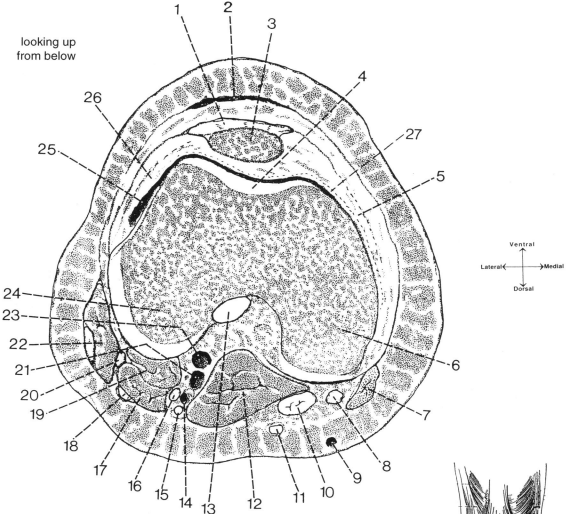

looking up
from below

after Ellis, Logan, and Dixon

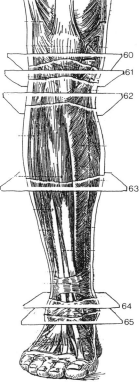

## SECTION 60
**Right Knee**

*Color and label:*

1. Patellar ligament (actually, tendon of quadriceps femoris)
2. Prepatellar bursa
3. Patella
4. Articular surface (cartilage) of femur
5. Medial patellar retinaculum
6. Medial condyle of femur
7. Sartorius muscle
8. Tendon of gracilis muscle
9. Great saphenous vein
10. Semimembranosus tendon
11. Semitendinosus tendon
12. Medial head of gastrocnemius muscle
13. Anterior cruciate ligament
14. Small saphenous vein
15. Sural nerve
16. Tibial nerve
17. Lateral head of gastrocnemius muscle
18. Sural communicating nerve
19. Plantaris muscle
20. Common peroneal (fibular) nerve
21. Popliteal vein
22. Biceps femoris muscle and tendon
23. Popliteal artery
24. Lateral femoral condyle
25. Articular cavity
26. Lateral patellar retinaculum and iliotibial tract
27. Capsule of joint cavity

*Fibula* **means "brooch" or "buckle" in Latin,** specifically the thin pointed tongue, as opposed to the much thicker and often highly ornate bar, of a clasp. Supposedly the Romans thought that the two bones of the lower leg resembled a clasp, with the outer thin bone suggesting the tongue and the inner thicker bone suggesting the bar. So they named the outer thin bone *fibula* and the inner thicker bone *tibia*. The term fibula probably arose from the verb *figo*—"to fix" or "fasten."

The muscles and structures on the outer side of the lower leg that relate to the fibula were named, not fibular as you might expect, but *peroneal* (Gr., *perone*—"brooch" derived from *peiro*—"to pierce"). Poorer Romans, who could not afford the metallic clasps or fibulae, most likely used the bones of animals to hold their clothes together.

It appears that most of the world's anatomists prefer fibular to peroneal as a name for these structures, and eventually we will see fibular completely replace peroneal. So instead of *peroneus longus* and *peroneus brevis*, these two muscles will become fibularis longus and fibularis brevis. An easy way to remember which is which is to recall that the fibula is lateral and the word fibula ends with **la** as in **la**teral.

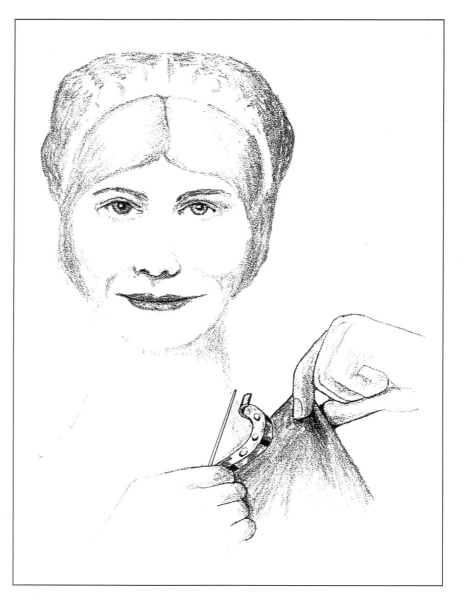

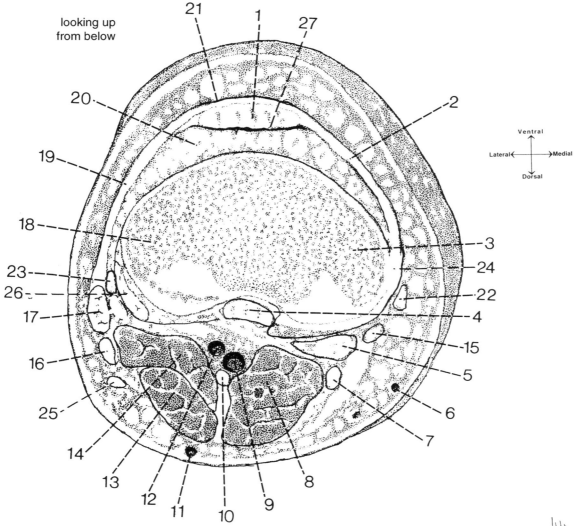

looking up
from below

Ventral
Lateral ← → Medial
Dorsal

*after Ellis, Logan, and Dixon*

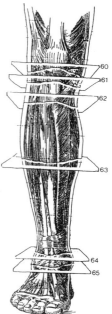

## SECTION 61
## Right Tibial Condyles

*Color and label:*

1. Patellar ligament
2. Medial patellar retinaculum
3. Medial condyle of tibia
4. Posterior cruciate ligament
5. Semimembranosus tendon
6. Great saphenous vein
7. Semitendinosus tendon
8. Gastrocnemius muscle, medial head
9. Popliteal vein
10. Tibial nerve
11. Small saphenous vein
12. Popliteal artery
13. Gastrocnemius muscle, lateral head
14. Plantaris muscle

15. Gracilis tendon
16. Common peroneal (fibular) nerve
17. Tendon of biceps femoris
18. Lateral tibial condyle
19. Lateral patellar retinaculum
20. Infrapatellar fat
21. Infrapatellar (subcutaneous) bursa
22. Sartorius tendon
23. Fibular (lateral) collateral ligament
24. Tibial (medial) collateral ligament
25. Lateral cutaneous nerve of calf
26. Popliteus muscle (tendinous origin)
27. Deep infrapatellar bursa

## Lateral Muscles
## of Right Leg

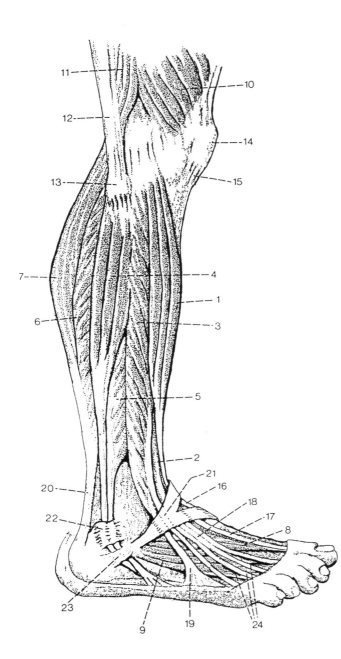

*after Clemente*

*Color and label (at left):*

1. Tibialis anterior
2. Extensor hallucis longus
3. Extensor digitorum longus
4. Fibularis longus (peroneus longus
5. Fibularis brevis (peroneus brevis)
6. Soleus
7. Gastrocnemius
8. Extensor hallucis brevis
9. Extensor digitorum brevis
10. Vastus lateralis
11. Biceps femoris
12. Tendon of biceps femoris
13. Head of fibula
14. Patella
15. Patellar ligament (actually tendon of quadriceps femoris)
16. Tendon of tibialis anterior
17. Tendon of extensor hallucis longus
18. Tendons of extensor digitorum longus
19. Tendon of fibularis tertius (peroneus tertius)
20. Tendo calcaneus (Achilles tendon)
21. Inferior extensor retinaculum
22. Superior fibular (peroneal) retinaculum
23. Inferior fibular (peroneal) retinaculum
24. Tendons of extensor digitorum brevis

## SECTION 62
## Right Lower Leg (Upper Part)

*Color and label (bottom):*

1. Tibia
2. Popliteus muscle
3. Soleus muscle
4. Medial head of gastrcnemius muscle
5. Posterior tibial vein
6. Tibial nerve
7. Posterior tibial artery
8. Peroneal artery
9. Lateral head of gastrocnemius muscle
10. Fibula
11. Superficial peroneal (fibular) nerve
12. Peroneus longus muscle
13. Deep peroneal nerve and anterior tibial artery
14. Extensor digitorum longus muscle
15. Tibialis posterior muscle
16. Tibialis anterior muscle
17. Interosseous membrane
18. Great saphenous vein and saphenous nerve
19. Lesser saphenous vein and sural nerve

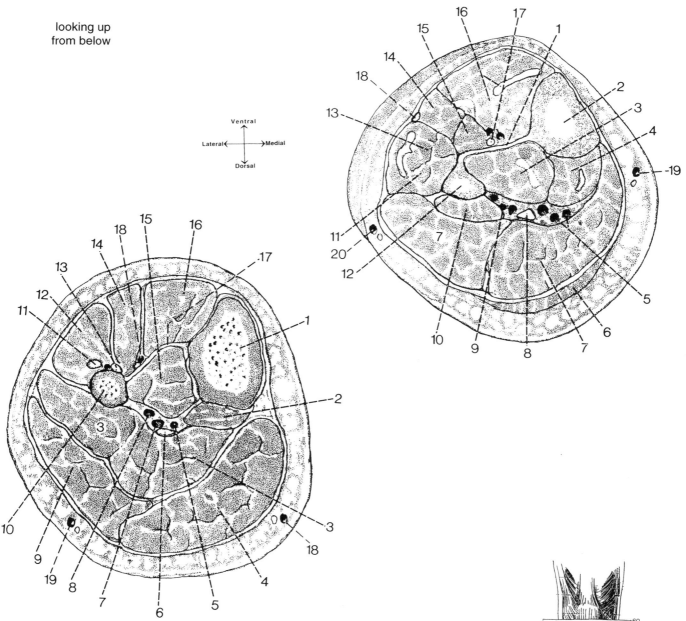

looking up
from below

Ventral
Lateral ← → Medial
Dorsal

*after Ellis, Logan, and Dixon*

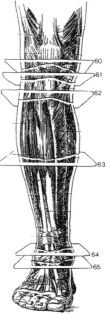

## SECTION 63
## Right Lower Leg (Mid Part)

*Color and label (top):*

1. Interosseous membrane
2. Tibia
3. Tibialis posterior muscle
4. Flexor digitorum longus muscle
5. Posterior tibial artery and vein
6. Gastrocnemius muscle
7. Soleus muscle
8. Tibial nerve
9. Peroneal artery and vein(s)
10. Flexor hallucis longus muscle
11. Peroneus longus muscle
12. Fibula

13. Peroneus brevis muscle
14. Extensor digitorum longus muscle
15. Extensor hallucis longus muscle
16. Tibialis anterior muscle and tendon
17. Deep peroneal nerve and
    anterior tibial artery and vein
18. Superficial peroneal nerve
19. Great saphenous vein
    and saphenous nerve
20. Lesser saphenous vein
    and sural nerve

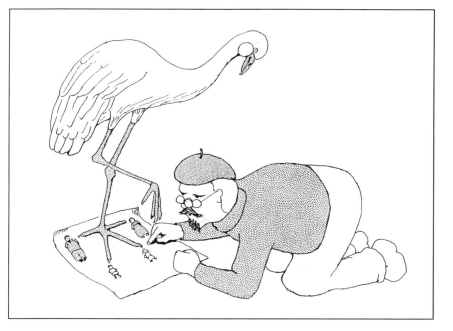

**The word for one's bloodline or pedigree involves the crane.** "Pedigree" is derived from the Latin "foot of the crane" (*pes, pedi*—"foot" + *de*—"of" + *grue*—"crane"). This came about because of the resemblance of a crane's foot to the lines of succession on a genealogical chart. So instead of saying "my family lineage," one would say "my family's *ped de grue* (foot of the crane)."

## SECTION 64
## Right Lower Leg (Lower Part)

*Color and label (bottom):*

1. Tibia
2. Saphenous nerve
3. Great saphenous vein
4. Tendon of tibialis posterior
5. Flexor digitorum longus muscle and tendon
6. Posterior tibial vein
7. Posterior tibial artery
8. Tibial nerve
9. Flexor hallucis longus muscle
10. Soleus muscle
11. Sural nerve
12. Small saphenous vein
13. Peroneus brevis muscle
14. Tendon of peroneus longus muscle
15. Fibula
16. Peroneal artery
17. Peroneus tertius muscle
18. Tendon of extensor digitorum longus muscle
19. Deep peroneal nerve
20. Anterior tibial artery
21. Tendon of tibialis anterior
22. Tendo calcaneus (Achilles tendon)
23. Tendon of extensor hallucis longus
24. Plantaris tendon

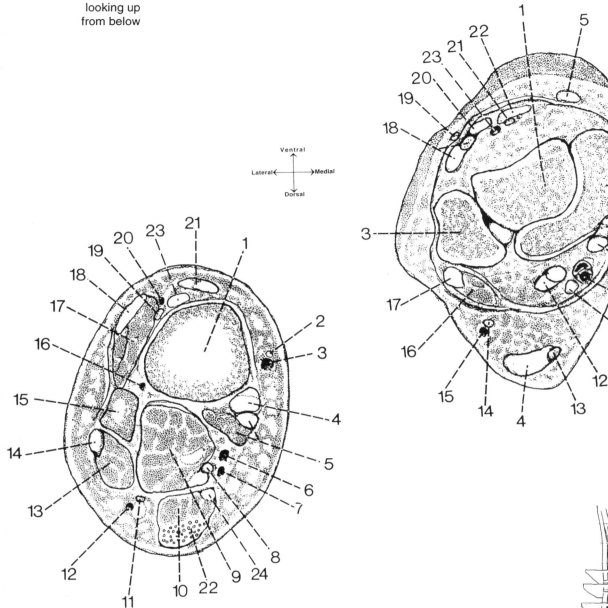

looking up
from below

Ventral
Lateral ← → Medial
Dorsal

*after Ellis, Logan, and Dixon*

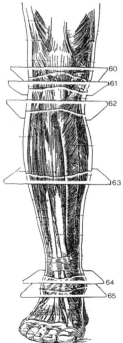

## SECTION 65
## Right Ankle

*Color and label (top):*

1. Talus (trochlea)
2. Medial malleolus of tibia
3. Lateral malleolus of fibula
4. Tendo calcaneus (Achilles tendon)
5. Tendon of tibialis anterior
6. Saphenous nerve
7. Great saphenous vein
8. Tendon of tibialis posterior
9. Tendon of flexor digitorum longus
10. Posterior tibial artery and vein(s)
11. Tibial nerve
12. Tendon of flexor hallucis longus

13. Tendon of plantaris
14. Sural nerve
15. Small saphenous vein
16. Peroneus brevis muscle
17. Tendon of peroneus longus
18. Peroneus tertius muscle and tendon
19. Superficial peroneal nerve
20. Tendon extensor digitorum longus
21. Deep peroneal nerve
22. Tendon of extensor hallucis longus
23. Anterior tibial artery

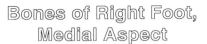

## Bones of Right Foot, Medial Aspect

level of
section 66

level of
section 67

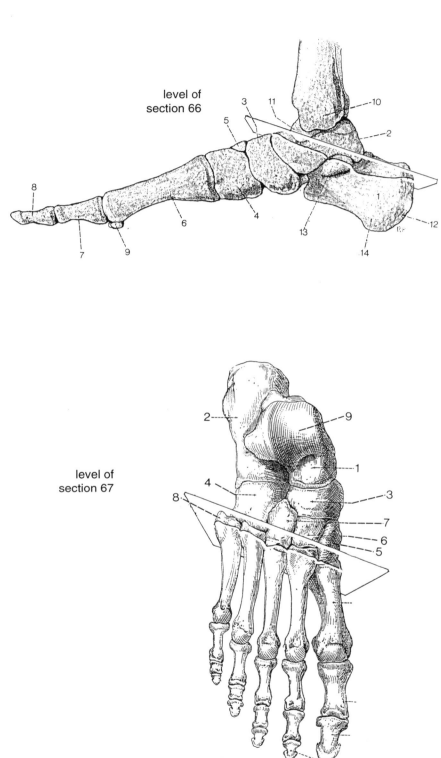

*after Eycleshymer and Jones*

*Color and label (left, top):*

1. Calcaneus
2. Talus
3. Navicular bone
4. Medial cuneiform bone
5. Intermediate cuneiform bone
6. First metatarsal bone
7. Proximal phalanx of big toe (hallux)
8. Distal phalanx of big toe
9. Sesamoid bones (in tendons of flexor hallucis brevis)
10. Medial malleolus (tibia)
11. Medial malleolar surface of talar trochlea
12. Tuberosity of calcaneus
13. Sustentaculum tali (of calcaneus)
14. Medial process of calcaneal tuberosity

*Color and label (left, bottom):*

1. Talus
2. Calcaneus
3. Navicular
4. Cuboid
5. Medial cuneiform
6. Intermediate cuneiform
7. Lateral cuneiform
8. Tuberosity on base of 5th metatarsal
9. Trochlea of talus

## SECTION 66
## Right Foot, Talus and Calcaneus

*Color and label (right, bottom):*

1. Talus
2. Tendon of extensor hallucis longus
3. Tendon of tibialis anterior
4. Great saphenous vein
5. Talocalcaneal joint
6. Tendon of tibialis posterior ("Tom")
7. Sustentaculum tali (part of calcaneus)
8. Tendon of flexor digitorum longus ("Dick")
9. Tendon of flexor hallucis longus ("Harry")
10. Medial plantar artery, vein, and nerve
11. Lateral plantar artery, vein, and nerve
12. Quadratus plantae muscle (also called flexor accessorius)
13. Calcaneal tuberosity
14. Tendo calcaneus (Achilles tendon)
15. Calcaneus
16. Tendon of peroneus longus
17. Tendon of peroneus brevis
18. Talus, lateral tuberosity (or process)
19. Talocalcaneal joint
20. Extensor digitorum brevis muscle
21. Tendons of extensor digitorum longus
22. Dorsalis pedis artery (continuation of anterior tibial artery)
23. Interosseous talocalcaneal ligament in tarsal sinus

viewed from
the front

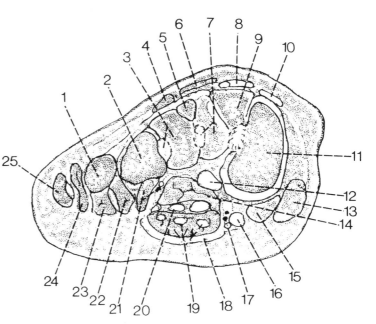

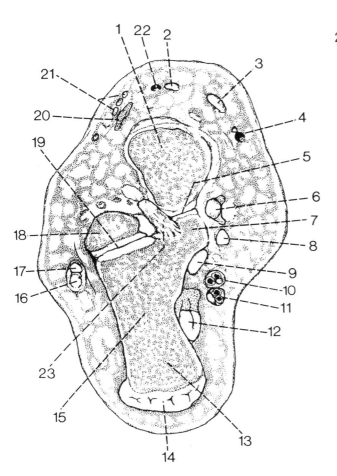

*after Ellis, Logan, and Dixon*

## SECTION 67
## Right Foot, Base of Metatarsals

*Color and label (top):*

1. Fifth metatarsal bone
2. Fourth metatarsal bone
3. Third metatarsal bone
   and interosseous ligament
4. Extensor digitorum brevis muscle
5. Lateral cuneiform (a small piece)
6. Tendon of extensor digitorum longus
7. Second metatarsal bone
   and interosseous ligament
8. Extensor hallucis brevis muscle
9. Medial cuneiform bone
10. Tendon of extensor hallucis longus
11. First metatarsal bone
12. Tendon of peroneus longus

13. Abductor hallucis muscle
14. Adductor hallucis muscle, oblique head
15. Flexor hallucis brevis muscle
16. Tendon of flexor hallucis longus
17. Medial plantar artery, vein, and nerve
18. Plantar aponeurosis
19. Flexor digitorum brevis muscle and tendons
20. Tendons of flexor digitorum longus muscle
21. Second plantar interosseous muscle
    and lateral plantar artery, vein, and nerve
22. Third plantar interosseous muscle
23. Flexor digiti minimi muscle
24. Opponens digiti minimi muscle
25. Abductor digiti minimi muscle

# Upper Extremity
## Sections 68 to 78

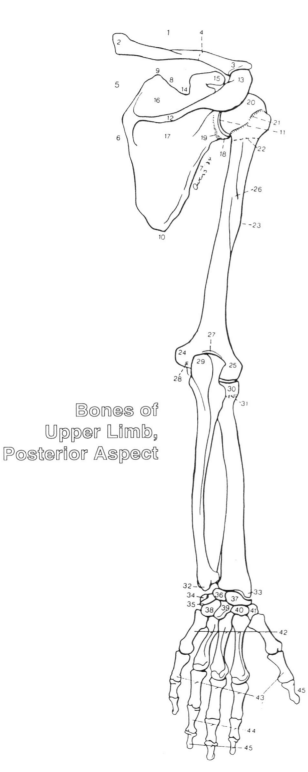

Bones of
Upper Limb,
Posterior Aspect

*Color and label (at left):*

1. Clavicle (collar bone)
2. Sternal (medial) end
3. Acromial (lateral) end
4. Most frequent site of fracture (clavicle is most frequently broken bone)
5. Scapula (shoulder blade)
6. Medial (vertebral) border
7. Lateral (axillary) border
8. Superior border
9. Superior angle
10. Inferior angle
11. Lateral angle (forms glenoid cavity)
12. Spine of scapula
13. Acromion
14. Scapular notch
15. Coracoid process
16. Supraspinatus fossa (for supraspinatus muscle)
17. Infraspinatus fossa (for infraspinatus muscle)
18. Infraglenoid tubercle (for triceps long head origin)
19. Neck of scapula
20. Head of humerus
21. Anatomical neck (rarely fractured)
22. Surgical neck (site of usual fracture at proximal humerus)
23. Deltoid tuberosity
24. Medial epicondyle
25. Lateral epicondyle
26. Radial groove for radial nerve
27. Olecranon fossa under olecranon
28. Sulcus for ulnar nerve
29. Olecranon
30. Head of radius
31. Neck of radius
32. Styloid process of ulna
33. Styloid process of radius
34. Pisiform bone
35. Triquetral bone
36. Lunate bone (most frequently dislocated wrist bone)
37. Scaphoid bone (most frequently fractured wrist bone)
38. Hamate bone
39. Capitate bone
40. Trapezoid bone
41. Trapezium bone
42. Metacarpal bones
43. Proximal phalanx
44. Middle phalanx
45. Distal phalanx

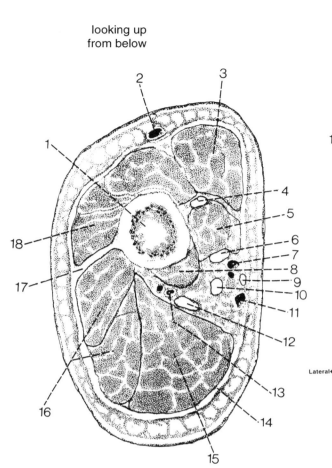

looking up
from below

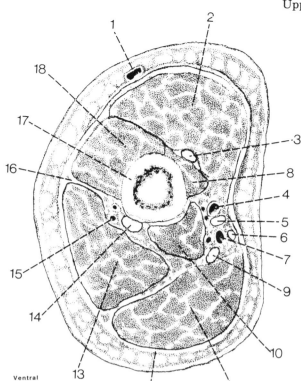

Ventral

Lateral ← → Medial

Dorsal

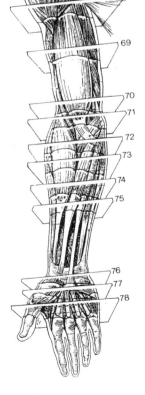

## SECTION 68
## Right Upper Arm*

*Color and label:*

1. Humerus (shaft)
2. Cephalic vein
3. Biceps brachii muscle
4. Musculocutaneous nerve
5. Coracobrachialis muscle
6. Median nerve
7. Brachial artery
8. Medial head of triceps brachii muscle
9. Medial antebrachial cutaneous nerve
10. Ulnar nerve
11. Brachial vein
12. Radial nerve
13. Profunda brachii artery and vein
14. Brachial fascia
15. Triceps brachii, long head
16. Triceps brachii, lateral head
17. Lateral intermuscular septum
18. Deltoid muscle

## SECTION 69
## Right Mid Arm

*Color and label:*

1. Cephalic vein
2. Biceps brachii muscle
3. Musculocutaneous nerve
4. Brachial artery
5. Median nerve
6. Medial antebrachial cutaneous nerve
7. Brachial vein
8. Coracobrachialis muscle
9. Ulnar nerve
10. Medial head of triceps brachii muscle
11. Long head of triceps brachii muscle
12. Brachial fascia
13. Lateral head of triceps brachii
14. Radial nerve
15. Profunda brachii artery and vein
16. Lateral intermuscular septum
17. Humerus (shaft)
18. Brachialis muscle

* In anatomy, the arm (Lat., brachium) extends from the shoulder to the elbow.
  The forearm (Lat., antebrachium) extends from the elbow to the wrist (Lat., carpus).

*after Eycleshymer and Jones*

## Superficial Forearm Dissection

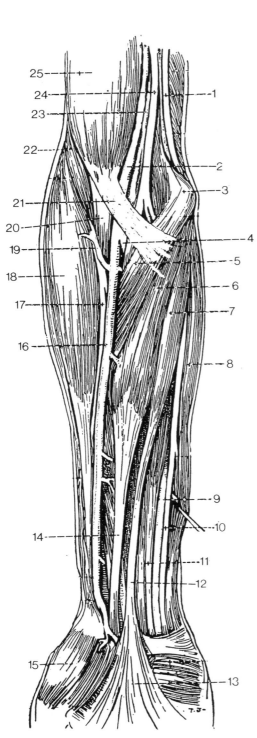

**Color and label (at left):**

1. Ulnar nerve
2. Brachial artery
3. Medial epicondyle of humerus
4. Ulnar artery (origin)
5. Pronator teres muscle
6. Flexor carpi radialis muscle
7. Palmaris longus muscle
8. Flexor carpi ulnaris muscle
9. Ulnar artery
10. Ulnar nerve
11. Tendon of flexor digitorum superficialis to 4th finger
12. Tendon of palmaris longus
13. Palmar aponeurosis
14. Tendon of flexor carpi radialis
15. Abductor pollicis brevis muscle
16. Radial artery
17. Radial nerve superficial branch
18. Brachioradialis muscle
19. Recurrent radial artery
20. Tendon of biceps brachii muscle
21. Bicipital aponeurosis
22. Brachialis muscle
23. Brachial artery
24. Median nerve
25. Biceps brachii muscle

*after Eycleshymer and Jones*

looking up
from below

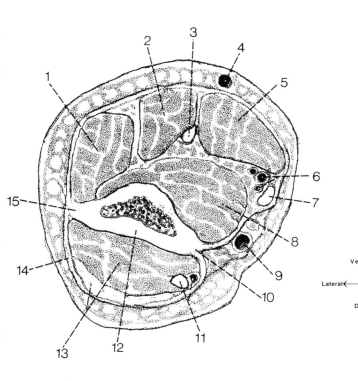

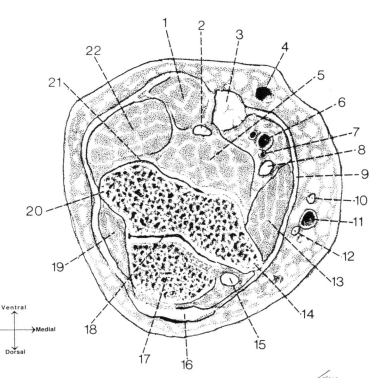

Ventral

Lateral ←→ Medial

Dorsal

## SECTION 70
## Right Lower Arm

*Color and label:*

1. Extensor carpi radialis longus muscle
2. Brachioradialis muscle
3. Radial nerve
4. Cephalic vein
5. Biceps brachii muscle
6. Brachial artery and brachial veins *
7. Median nerve
8. Brachialis muscle
9. Basilic vein
10. Medial epicondyle of humerus
11. Ulnar nerve and superior ulnar collateral artery
12. Shaft of humerus
13. Triceps brachii muscle and tendon
14. Brachial fascia
15. Lateral epicondyle of humerus

\* Veins that run with arteries are *venae comitantes*.

## SECTION 71
## Right Elbow

*Color and label:*

1. Brachioradialis muscle
2. Radial nerve
3. Tendon of biceps brachii
4. Cephalic vein
5. Brachialis muscle
6. Brachial artery
7. Brachial vein
8. Median nerve
9. Brachial fascia
10. Branch of medial antebrachial cutaneous nerve (divided)
11. Basilic vein
12. Branch of medial antebrachial cutaneous nerve
13. Pronator teres muscle
14. Medial epicondyle of humerus
15. Ulnar nerve ("funny bone")
16. Tendon of triceps brachii
17. Olecranon of ulna (tip of elbow)
18. Elbow joint (between trochlea of humerus and trochlear notch of ulna)
19. Anconeus muscle
20. Lateral epicondyle of humerus
21. Capitulum of humerus (lateral condyle)
22. Extensor carpi radials longus muscle

# Deep Forearm Dissection

*after Eycleshymer and Jones*

Color and label (at left):

1. Median nerve
2. Ulnar nerve
3. Medial epicondyle
4. Common origin of flexor muscles and pronator teres
5. Muscular branches of median nerve
6. Bicipital aponeurosis
7. Ulnar artery
8. Flexor digitorum profundus muscle
9. Tendon of flexor carpi radialis (cut)
10. Tendon of palmaris longus (cut)
11. Pronator quadratus muscle
12. Flexor pollicis longus muscle
13. Anterior interosseous artery
14. Superficial branch of radial nerve
15. Radial artery
16. Brachioradialis muscle
17. Deep branch of radial nerve
18. Tendon of biceps brachii
19. Radial nerve
20. Biceps brachii muscle
21. Brachial vein
22. Brachial artery

## SECTION 72
## Right Elbow

Color and label (bottom):

1. Brachioradialis muscle
2. Radial nerve
3. Tendon of biceps brachii muscle
4. Cephalic vein
5. Brachial artery and vein
6. Antebrachial fascia
7. Median nerve
8. Pronator teres muscle
9. Brachialis muscle
10. Trochlea of humerus (medial condyle of humerus)
11. Flexor carpi radialis muscle
12. Flexor digitorum superficialis muscle
13. Basilic vein
14. Ulnar nerve
15. Superior ulnar collateral artery and vein
16. Elbow joint (between trochlea of humerus and trochlear notch of ulna)
17. Ulna and coronoid process of ulna
18. Superior radio-ulnar joint (between head of radius and radial notch of ulna)
19. Anconeus muscle
20. Head of radius
21. Annular ligament
22. Extensor carpi radialis brevis muscle
23. Extensor carpi radialis longus muscle
24. Flexor carpi ulnaris muscle
25. Palmaris longus muscle

looking up
from below

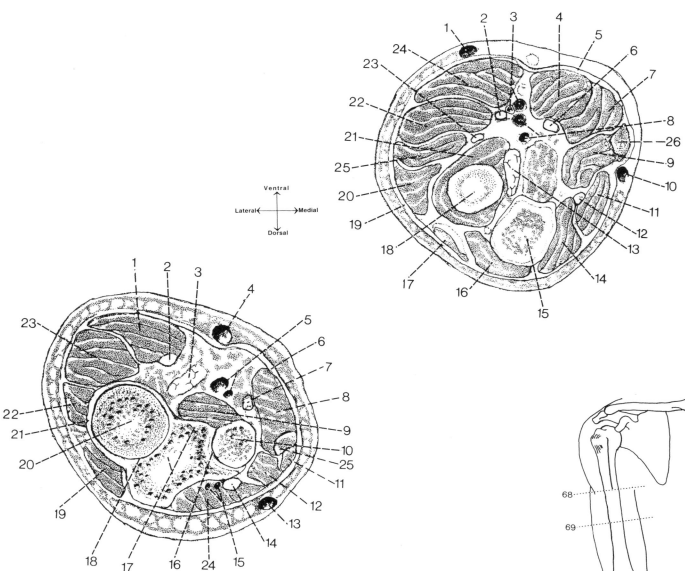

Ventral
Lateral← →Medial
Dorsal

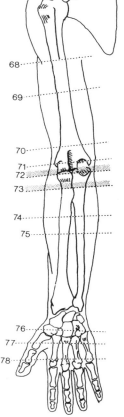

**SECTION 73**
**Right Upper Forearm**

*Color and label (top):*

1. Cephalic vein
2. Superficial branch of radial nerve
3. Radial artery and vein
4. Pronator teres
5. Antebrachial fascia
6. Median nerve
7. Flexor carpi radialis muscle
8. Ulnar artery and vein
9. Flexor digitorum superficialis muscle
10. Basilic vein
11. Flexor carpi ulnaris
12. Ulnar nerve
13. Biceps brachii tendon
14. Flexor digitorum profundus muscle
15. Ulna (shaft)
16. Anconeus muscle
17. Extensor carpi ulnaris muscle
18. Neck of radius
19. Antebrachial fascia
20. Extensor digitorum muscle
21. Supinator muscle
22. Extensor carpi radialis longus muscle
23. Deep branch of radial nerve
24. Brachioradialis muscle
25. Extensor carpi radialis brevis muscle
26. Palmaris longus muscle

## Muscles of Arm, Lateral Aspect

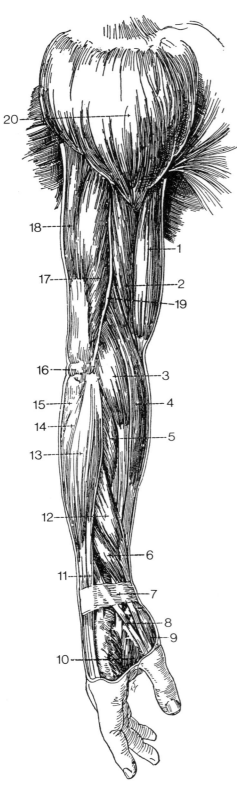

*Color and label (at left):*

1. Biceps brachii muscle
2. Brachialis muscle
3. Extensor carpi radialis longus muscle
4. Brachioradialis muscle
5. Extensor carpi radialis brevis muscle
6. Extensor pollicis brevis muscle
7. "Snuff box"
8. Tendon of extensor pollicis longus
9. Thenar muscles
10. First dorsal interosseous muscle (note its two heads)
11. Tendons of extensor digitorum
12. Abductor pollicis longus muscle
13. Extensor digitorum muscle
14. Extensor carpi ulnaris muscle
15. Anconeus muscle
16. Olecranon (bony tip of elbow)
17. Triceps brachii lateral head
18. Triceps brachii long head
19. Lateral intermuscular septum
20. Deltoid muscle

*after Eycleshymer and Jones*

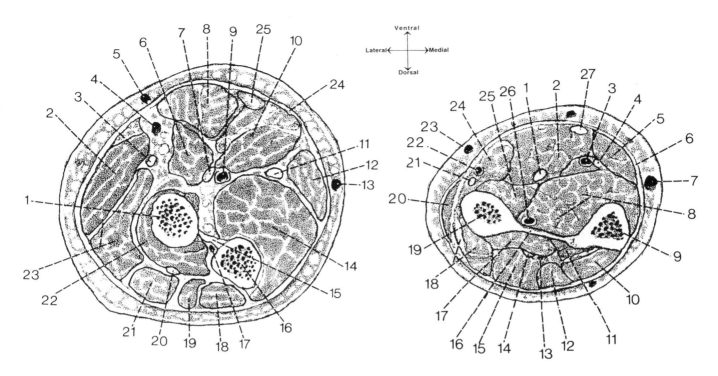

looking up from below

Ventral
Lateral ←→ Medial
Dorsal

## SECTION 74
### Right Mid Forearm

*Color and label:*

1. Radius (shaft)
2. Brachioradialis muscle
3. Superficial branch of radial nerve
4. Radial artery
5. Cephalic vein
6. Pronator teres muscle
7. Median nerve
8. Flexor carpi radialis muscle
9. Ulnar artery
10. Flexor digitorum superficialis muscle
11. Ulnar nerve
12. Flexor carpi ulnaris muscle
13. Basilic vein
14. Flexor digitorum profundus muscle
15. Interosseous membrane
16. Ulna (shaft)
17. Posterior interosseous artery
18. Extensor carpi ulnaris muscle
19. Extensor digiti minimi muscle
20. Deep branch of radial nerve
21. Extensor digitorum muscle
22. Supinator muscle
23. Extensor carpi radialis longus (tendon) and extensor carpi radialis brevis muscle
24. Antebrachial fascia
25. Palmaris longus muscle

## SECTION 75
### Right Lower Forearm

*Color and label:*

1. Median nerve
2. Flexor digitorum superficialis muscle
3. Ulnar artery
4. Ulnar nerve
5. Flexor carpi ulnaris muscle
6. Antebrachial fascia
7. Basilic vein
8. Flexor digitorum profundus
9. Ulna (shaft)
10. Extensor carpi ulnaris muscle
11. Extensor pollicis longus muscle
12. Extensor digiti minimi muscle
13. Posterior interosseous artery (off common interosseous artery)
14. Deep branch of radial nerve
15. Extensor digitorum muscle
16. Interosseous membrane
17. Abductor pollicis longus muscle
18. Extensor carpi radialis longus (tendon) and extensor carpi radialis brevis muscle
19. Radius (shaft)
20. Brachioradialis muscle
21. Superficial branch of radial nerve
22. Radial artery
23. Cephalic vein
24. Flexor carpi radialis muscle
25. Flexor pollicis longus muscle
26. Anterior interosseous artery (off common interosseous artery)
27. Tendon of palmaris longus muscle

## Hand, Dissected

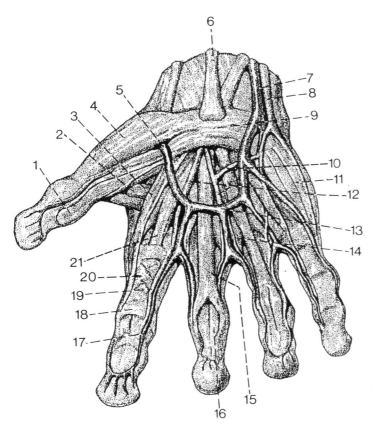

**oblique view, palmar aspect**
**skin and palmar aponeurosis removed**

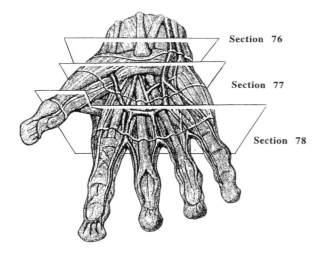

*Color and label (at left):*

1. Tendon of flexor pollicis longus muscle
2. Adductor pollicis muscle
3. First lumbrical muscle
4. Abductor pollicis muscle
5. Radial artery
6. Cut end of tendon of palmaris longus
7. Ulnar artery
8. Ulnar nerve
9. Flexor retinaculum
10. Communicating branch of ulnar with median nerve
11. Hypothenar muscles
12. Common palmar digital branches of median nerve
13. Superficial palmar (arterial) arch
14. Common palmar digital nerve and artery
15. Tendon of flexor digitorum superficialis muscle to 3rd finger
16. Tendon of flexor digitorum profundus
17. Proper palmar digital artery
18. Annular fibers of fibrous tendon sheath
19. Proper palmar digital nerve
20. Cruciate fibers of fibrous tendon sheath
21. Tendon of flexor digitorum superficialis muscle

## SECTION 76
## Wrist Level

*Color and label (right, bottom):*

1. Flexor retinaculum (forms "roof" or ventral wall of carpal tunnel
2. Ulnar artery
3. Ulnar nerve
4. Four tendons of flexor digitorum superficialis muscle
5. Hypothenar muscles
6. Hook (uncus) of hamate bone
7. Four tendons of flexor digitorum profundus muscle
8. Tendon of extensor carpi ulnaris muscle
9. Tendon of extensor digiti minimi muscle
10. Hamate bone (carpal bone)
11. Tendons of extensor digitorum muscle
12. Capitate bone (carpal bone)
13. Tendon of extensor indicis
14. Tendon of extensor carpi radialis brevis
15. Trapezoid bone (carpal bone)
16. Tendon of extensor carpi radialis longus muscle
17. Tendon of extensor pollicis longus muscle
18. Radial artery (in snuff box)
19. Cephalic vein
20. Trapezium (carpal bone)
21. Tendon of extensor pollicis brevis muscle
22. Tendon of abductor pollicis longus muscle
23. Opponens pollicis muscle
24. Tendon of flexor carpi radialis muscle
25. Tendon of flexor pollicis longus muscle
26. Abductor pollicis brevis muscle
27. Median nerve
28. Flexor pollicis brevis muscle
29. "Snuff box"

looking up
from below

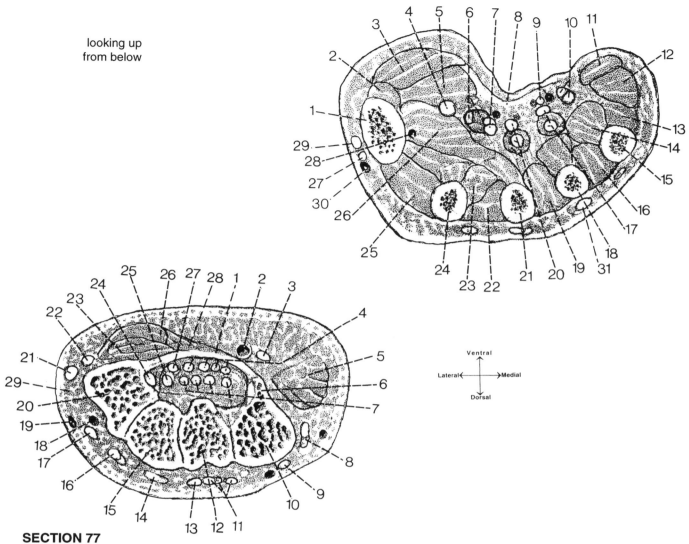

Ventral
Lateral ← → Medial
Dorsal

**SECTION 77**
**Right Hand**

*Color and label (top):*

1. First metacarpal bone
2. Opponens pollicis muscle
3. Abductor pollicis brevis muscle
4. Tendon of flexor pollicis longus muscle
5. Flexor pollicis brevis muscle
6. Median nerve and first lumbrical muscle
7. Tendons of flexor digitorum superficialis and flexor digitorum profundus to index finger
8. Palmar aponeurosis
9. Ulnar nerve and arterial branch off superficial palmar arch
10. Superficial and deep flexor tendons to fifth finger
11. Flexor digiti minimi muscle
12. Abductor digiti minimi muscle
13. Opponens digiti minimi muscle
14. Ventral (palmar or volar) interosseous muscle
15. Fifth metacarpal bone
16. Fourth dorsal interosseous muscle
17. Tendons of superficial flexor muscle and deep (profundus) flexor muscle to 4th digit (deep tendon is surrounded by third lumbrical muscle)
18. Fourth metacarpal bone
19. Third dorsal interosseous muscle
20. Tendons of superficial and deep flexor muscles to third finger (deep tendon is surrounded by second lumbrical muscle)
21. Third metacarpal bone
22. Second dorsal interosseous muscle
23. First ventral (palmar or volar) interosseous muscle
24. Second metacarpal bone
25. First dorsal interosseous muscle
26. Adductor pollicis muscle
27. Cephalic vein
28. Radial artery
29. Tendon of extensor pollicis brevis
30. Tendon of extensor pollicis longus
31. Tendon of extensor digitorum to 4th digit

# Arteries of Thorax and Arm

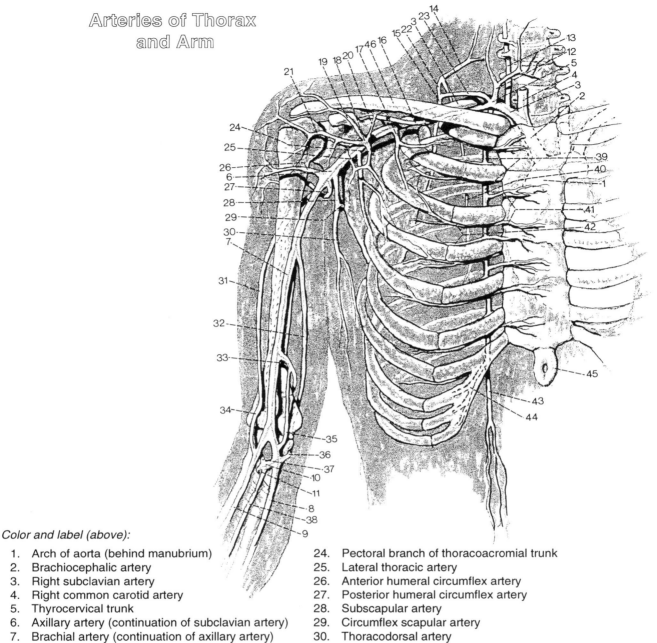

*Color and label (above):*

1. Arch of aorta (behind manubrium)
2. Brachiocephalic artery
3. Right subclavian artery
4. Right common carotid artery
5. Thyrocervical trunk
6. Axillary artery (continuation of subclavian artery)
7. Brachial artery (continuation of axillary artery)
8. Ulnar artery
9. Radial artery
10. Common interosseous artery
11. Posterior interosseous artery
12. Inferior thyroid artery
13. Vertebral artery
14. Ascending branch of superficial branch of transverse cervical artery
15. Deep branch of transverse cervical artery
16. Suprascapular artery
17. Supreme thoracic artery
18. Thoracoacromial trunk
19. Acromial branch of thoracoacromial trunk
20. Clavicular branch
21. Deltoid branch
22. Superficial branch of transverse cervical artery
23. Transverse cervical artery

24. Pectoral branch of thoracoacromial trunk
25. Lateral thoracic artery
26. Anterior humeral circumflex artery
27. Posterior humeral circumflex artery
28. Subscapular artery
29. Circumflex scapular artery
30. Thoracodorsal artery
31. Radial collateral artery of deep brachial artery
32. Superior ulnar collateral artery
33. Inferior ulnar collateral artery
34. Radial recurrent artery
35. Anterior ulnar recurrent artery
36. Posterior ulnar recurrent artery
37. Recurrent interosseous artery
38. Anterior interosseous artery
39. Internal thoracic artery
40. Descending branch of superficial branch of transverse cervical artery
41. Perforating branches of internal thoracic artery
42. Anterior intercostal arteries
43. Superior epigastric artery
44. Musculophrenic artery
45. Xiphoid process
46. Deep (profunda) brachial artery (behind humerus)

looking up
from below

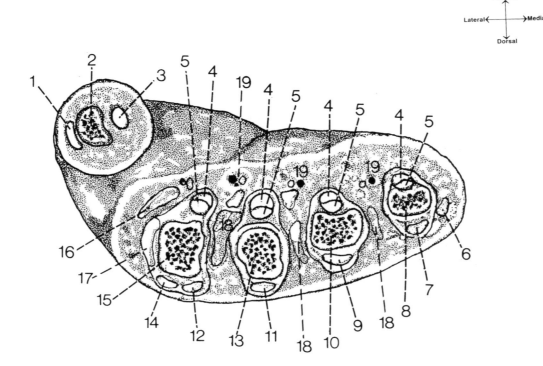

Ventral

Lateral ← → Medial

Dorsal

## SECTION 78
### Right Hand

*Color and label:*

1. Tendon of extensor pollicis longus
2. Distal phalanx of thumb
3. Tendon of flexor pollicis longus
4. Superficial flexor tendons to digits 2–5
5. Deep flexor tendons to digits 2–5
6. Tendon of extensor digiti minimi
7. Extensor digitorum tendon to fifth finger
8. Fifth metacarpal
9. Extensor digitorum tendon to fourth finger
10. Fourth metacarpal bone

11. Extensor digitorum tendon to third finger
12. Extensor indicis tendon to second finger
13. Third metacarpal
14. Extensor digitorum tendon to second (index) finger
15. Second metacarpal
16. First lumbrical muscle
17. First dorsal interosseous muscle
18. Compartments for interosseous muscles
19. Neurovascular bundles to each finger